50 SYMPTOMS OF MENOPAUSE

Understanding and Navigating the Menopausal Transition

Copyright, Menopause Matter 2023
All Rights Reserved. No part of this book can be reproduced without the written permission of the publisher.
Cover Designed by Samiahmed321
Edited by Heather Desna
Published by COJ Bookz

Dedication

Thank you to The Black Business initiative for believing in our cause.
Menopause affects a significant portion of the population and can have a profound impact on women's health and well-being.

By supporting Menopause Matter, we can help raise awareness about the importance of women's health during this transition and improve the quality of life for women experiencing menopause.

Table Of Contents

Introduction 1
50 Symptom of Peri Menopause, Menopause, Post Menopause 2
What is Perimenopause? 2
What is Menopause? 3
What is Post Menopause? 4
50 Symptoms of Menopause 5
Symptoms 7
Ways to Alleviate Symptoms 15
Menopause and Your Career 55
Menopause and Relationships 57
Foods To Avoid During Menopause 58
Journalling During Menopause 59
How To Prepare for Bedtime During Menopause 60
What is HRT Hormone Replacement Therapy 61
Snoring and Menopause 62
Foods to eat during Menopause 67
Exercises to do during Menopause 71
Black Women and Menopause 73
References 75

Introduction

As women approach midlife, they enter a new phase of life marked by profound physical, emotional, and hormonal changes. Menopause, the cessation of menstrual periods, can bring on a host of symptoms that affect women's daily lives in many ways. From hot flashes and night sweats to mood swings and fatigue, menopause can be a challenging time for many women.

Despite its ubiquity, menopause remains a taboo topic in many cultures, leaving women feeling isolated and unsupported.

This book aims to change that. We have compiled a comprehensive guide to the 50 most common symptoms of menopause, providing detailed information on the causes and effects of each symptom, as well as natural remedies and coping strategies that women can use to manage their symptoms. Our hope is that this book will serve as a valuable resource for women experiencing menopause, as well as for their partners and families. We believe that by providing accurate, accessible information on menopause, we can help women navigate this important phase of life with confidence, strength, and grace.

All Proceeds from the sale of this book goes towards programs, workshops and fundraising for Menopause Matter.

50 Symptom of Peri Menopause, Menopause, Post Menopause

What is Perimenopause?

Perimenopause is caused by a gradual decline in the production of estrogen and progesterone by the ovaries. As a woman approaches her late 30s and 40s, her ovaries begin to produce less estrogen and progesterone, which can cause changes in her menstrual cycle and other symptoms associated with perimenopause.

The decline in hormone production is a natural part of the aging process and is influenced by a number of factors, including genetics, lifestyle, and environmental factors. Some women may experience perimenopause earlier than others due to factors such as smoking, exposure to toxins, and certain medical conditions that can affect the ovaries.

Perimenopause can also be influenced by other hormonal factors, such as changes in levels of follicle-stimulating hormone (FSH) and luteinizing hormone (LH), which are produced by the pituitary gland in response to declining estrogen levels.

In some cases, medical treatments such as chemotherapy or radiation therapy can also cause premature perimenopause or menopause by damaging the ovaries. Additionally, some surgical procedures such as hysterectomy or oophorectomy (removal of the ovaries) can also cause perimenopause to occur earlier than it would have naturally.

What is Menopause?

Menopause is a natural biological process that marks the end of a woman's reproductive years. It is diagnosed when a woman has not had a menstrual period for 12 consecutive months.

Menopause typically occurs between the ages of 45 and 55, but it can occur earlier or later.

The cause of menopause is the decline in the production of estrogen and progesterone by the ovaries. As a woman ages, her ovaries gradually produce less estrogen and progesterone, which can cause changes in her menstrual cycle and other symptoms associated with menopause.

The decline in hormone production is a natural part of the aging process and is influenced by a number of factors, including genetics, lifestyle, and environmental factors. Some women may experience menopause earlier than others due to factors such as smoking, exposure to toxins, and certain medical conditions that can affect the ovaries.

In addition to the decline in estrogen and progesterone production, menopause can also be influenced by other hormonal factors, such as changes in levels of follicle-stimulating hormone (FSH) and luteinizing hormone (LH), which are produced by the pituitary gland in response to declining estrogen levels.

In some cases, medical treatments such as chemotherapy or radiation therapy can also cause premature menopause by damaging the ovaries. Additionally, some surgical procedures such as hysterectomy or oophorectomy (removal of the ovaries) can also cause menopause to occur earlier than it would have naturally

What is Post Menopause?

Post menopause is the stage of a woman's reproductive life that occurs after menopause, which is diagnosed when a woman has not had a menstrual period for 12 consecutive months. Post menopause is a natural part of the aging process and lasts for the rest of a woman's life.

The cause of post menopause is the permanent decline in the production of estrogen and progesterone by the ovaries. After menopause, the ovaries no longer produce eggs, and the level of hormones in a woman's body remains low for the rest of her life.

The decline in hormone production can cause changes in a woman's body that increase the risk of certain health conditions, such as osteoporosis, heart disease, and vaginal dryness. It is important for women to take steps to maintain their health and reduce their risk of these conditions during post menopause.

50 Symptoms of Menopause

- Irregular periods
- Hot flashes
- Night sweats
- Vaginal dryness
- Decreased libido
- Mood swings
- Depression
- Anxiety
- Insomnia
- Fatigue
- Weight gain
- Bloating
- Headaches
- Joint pain
- Muscle tension
- Memory lapses
- Difficulty concentrating
- Brain fog
- Hair loss or thinning
- Dry skin
- Acne
- Brittle nails
- Breast tenderness
- Itchy skin
- Allergies
- Dry eyes
- Vision changes
- Tinnitus
- Dizziness
- Vertigo
- Heart palpitations
- High blood pressure
- Rapid heart rate
- Shortness of breath
- Chest pain
- Digestive problems
- Constipation
- Diarrhea

- Incontinence
- Urinary tract infections
- Yeast infections
- Oral health problems
- Gum disease
- Tooth decay
- Osteoporosis
- Arthritis
- Chronic fatigue syndrome
- Fibromyalgia
- Cancer (breast, ovarian, or endometrial)
- Diabetes

It's important to note that not all women will experience all of these symptoms, and the severity and duration of symptoms can vary widely among women. If you're experiencing symptoms of menopause, talk to your healthcare provider about your options for managing them.

Symptoms

Irregular periods:

Menopause causes a decrease in estrogen production, which can cause menstrual cycles to become irregular. Women may experience missed periods, heavier or lighter bleeding, or longer or shorter cycles. These changes occur as the ovaries stop releasing eggs, and can last for several months to a few years before periods stop completely.

Hot flashes:

Hot flashes are a sudden sensation of intense heat that spreads throughout the body, often accompanied by sweating and flushing. They are caused by changes in estrogen levels, which affect thebody's ability to regulate temperature. Hot flashes can occur several times a day or night, and may last for several minutes to an hour.

Night sweats:

Night sweats are hot flashes that occur during sleep, and can cause sweating, chills, and disrupted sleep. They can lead to fatigue, mood changes, and difficulty concentrating during the day.

Vaginal dryness:

Menopause can cause the tissues of the vulva and vagina to become thin, dry, and less elastic. This can cause discomfort, itching, burning, and pain during intercourse. Women may also be at increased risk of urinary tract infections and other vaginal infections.

Decreased libido:

Menopause can cause a decrease in the hormone testosterone, which can affect sexual desire and function. Women may experience decreased interest in sex, difficulty becoming aroused, and decreased vaginal lubrication.

Mood swings:

Hormonal changes during menopause can cause mood swings, irritability, anxiety, and depression. These symptoms may be caused by changes in estrogen and progesterone levels, which affect the levels of neurotransmitters in the brain.

Depression:

Menopause is associated with an increased risk of depression, which may be caused by hormonal changes, stress, or other life changes. Symptoms of depression can include sadness, hopelessness, lack of interest in activities, changes in appetite, and difficulty sleeping

Anxiety:

Anxiety Is a common symptom of menopause, and may be caused by hormonal changes, stress, or other factors. Women may experience excessive worry, restlessness, panic attacks, and physical symptoms such as sweating, palpitations, and difficulty breathing.

Insomnia:

Menopause can cause difficulty falling asleep or staying asleep, which can lead to fatigue, irritability, and difficulty concentrating during the day. Insomnia may be caused by hot flashes, anxiety, or other factors.

Fatigue:

Many women experience fatigue during menopause, which can be caused by hormonal changes, sleep disturbances, or other factors. Fatigue can lead to difficulty concentrating, irritability, and decreased quality of life.

Weight gain:

Menopause is associated with an increase in body weight, particularly around the waist and hips. This may be caused by hormonal changes, decreased activity levels, and changes in metabolism

Bloating:

Bloating is a common symptom of menopause, and may be caused by hormonal changes, changes in digestion, or other factors. Women may experience abdominal discomfort, gas, and distention.

Headaches:

Menopause may be associated with an increase in headaches, including migraines. Hormonal changes, stress, and other factors may contribute to these symptoms.

Joint pain:

Menopause is associated with an increase in joint pain and stiffness, particularly in the hands, wrists, and knees. Hormonal changes, inflammation, and changes in activity levels may contribute to these symptoms.

Muscle tension:

Menopause may be associated with an increase in muscle tension, particularly in the neck, shoulders, and back. Hormonal changes, stress, and changes in activity levels may contribute to these symptoms.

Memory lapses:

Menopause may be associated with memory lapses, forgetfulness, and difficulty concentrating. These symptoms may be caused by hormonal changes, stress, or other factors.

Difficulty concentrating:

Menopause may affect cognitive function and cause difficulty concentrating, forgetfulness, and brain fog. These symptoms may be caused by hormonal changes, sleep disturbances, or other factors.

Brain fog:

Brain fog is a common symptom of menopause, and may be characterized by difficulty concentrating, forgetfulness, and confusion. Hormonal changes, stress, and other factors may contribute to these symptoms.

Hair loss or thinning:

Menopause can cause hair loss or thinning, particularly around the crown and temples. This may be caused by hormonal changes, genetics, or other factors.

Dry skin:

Menopause can cause dry, itchy skin, particularly on the face, neck, and hands. Hormonal changes decreased collagen production, and changes in oil production may contribute to these symptoms.

Acne:

Menopause may be associated with an increase in acne, particularly on the face and chin. Hormonal changes, stress, and other factors may contribute to these symptoms.

Brittle nails:

Menopause can cause nails to become brittle and weak, which may be caused by hormonal changes or nutrient deficiencies.

Breast tenderness:

Menopause may be associated with breast tenderness, swelling, and discomfort. Hormonal changes, fibrocystic breast changes, and other factors may contribute to these symptoms.

Itchy skin:

Menopause can cause dry, itchy skin, particularly on the face, neck, and hands. Hormonal changes decreased collagen production, and changes in oil production may contribute to these symptoms.

Allergies:

Menopause may be associated with an increase in allergies, particularly to environmental allergens such as pollen and dust. Hormonal changes and other factors may contribute to these symptoms.

Dry eyes:

Menopause can cause dry eyes, which may be caused by hormonal changes or other factors. Women may experience burning, itching, or blurred vision.

Vision changes:

Menopause may be associated with changes in vision, including difficulty seeing at night, blurred vision, and dry eyes. Hormonal changes, changes in tear production, and other factors may contribute to these symptoms.

Tinnitus:

Menopause may be associated with tinnitus, a ringing or buzzing in the ears. Hormonal changes, stress, and other factors may contribute to these symptoms.

Dizziness:

Menopause may be associated with dizziness, which may be caused by hormonal changes, changes in blood pressure, or other factors.

Vertigo:

Menopause may be associated with vertigo, a feeling of dizziness or spinning. Hormonal changes, changes in blood pressure, or other factors may contribute to these symptoms.

Heart palpitations:

Menopause may be associated with heart palpitations, which are a sensation of fluttering or racing in the chest. Hormonal changes, anxiety, and other factors may contribute to these symptoms.

High blood pressure:

Menopause may be associated with an increase in blood pressure, which can increase the risk of heart disease and other health problems.

Rapid heart rate:

Menopause may be associated with a rapid heart rate, which can cause palpitations, chest pain, and other symptoms. Hormonal changes, anxiety, and other factors may contribute to these symptoms.

Shortness of breath:

Menopause may be associated with shortness of breath, which can be caused by hormonal changes, anxiety, or other factors.

Chest pain:

Menopause may be associated with chest pain or discomfort, which can be caused by hormonal changes, heart disease, or other factors.

Digestive problems:

Menopause may be associated with digestive problems, such as bloating, constipation, or diarrhea. These symptoms may be caused by hormonal changes

Constipation:

Menopause may be associated with constipation, which can be caused by hormonal changes, decreased activity levels, or other factors.

Diarrhea:

Menopause may be associated with diarrhea, which can be caused by hormonal changes, changes in diet, or other factors.

Incontinence:

Menopause may be associated with incontinence, or the loss of bladder control. This may be caused by hormonal changes, changes in the pelvic floor muscles, or other factors.

Urinary tract infections:

Menopause may increase the risk of urinary tract infections (UTIs), which can cause painful urination, frequent urination, and other symptoms. This may be caused by changes in the urinary tract, decreased estrogen levels, or other factors.

Yeast infections:

Menopause may increase the risk of yeast infections, which can cause itching, burning, and discharge. This may be caused by hormonal changes, decreased estrogen levels, or other factors.

Oral health problems:

Menopause may increase the risk of oral health problems, such as dry mouth, gum disease, and tooth decay. This may be caused by hormonal changes, decreased saliva production, or other factors.

Gum disease:

Menopause may increase the risk of gum disease, which can cause inflammation, bleeding, and tooth loss. This may be caused by hormonal changes, decreased saliva production, or other factors.

Tooth decay:

Menopause may increase the risk of tooth decay, which can cause cavities and tooth loss. This may be caused by hormonal changes, decreased saliva production, or other factors.

Osteoporosis:

Menopause may increase the risk of osteoporosis, a condition in which bones become weak and brittle. This may be caused by decreased estrogen levels, changes in bone metabolism, or other factors.

Arthritis:

Menopause may increase the risk of arthritis, a condition that causes joint pain, stiffness, and swelling. This may be caused by hormonal changes, inflammation, or other factors.

Chronic fatigue syndrome:

Menopause may increase the risk of chronic fatigue syndrome, a condition characterized by extreme fatigue that is not relieved by rest. This may be caused by hormonal changes, immune system dysfunction, or other factors.

Fibromyalgia:

Menopause may increase the risk of fibromyalgia, a condition characterized by widespread pain, fatigue, and other symptoms. This may be caused by hormonal changes, stress, or other factors.

Cancer (breast, ovarian, or endometrial):

Menopause may increase the risk of certain types of cancer, including breast, ovarian, and endometrial cancer. This may be caused by hormonal changes, genetics, or other factors.

Diabetes:

Menopause may increase the risk of diabetes, a condition characterized by high blood sugar levels. This may be caused by hormonal changes, changes in metabolism, or other factors.

Ways to Alleviate Symptoms

Irregular periods:

Natural remedies such as black cohosh, red clover, and soy isoflavones have been found to help regulate menstrual cycles. Vitamin D and calcium supplements can also help improve bone health and reduce the risk of osteoporosis.

Black cohosh is a herb that has been shown to help regulate menstrual cycles. Red clover contains phytoestrogens, which can also help regulate periods. Soy isoflavones have been found to improve bone density and reduce hot flashes, which can be a beneficial side effect for women experiencing irregular periods.

Here is a list of natural remedies that may help with irregular periods:

Ginger: Ginger has been found to have anti-inflammatory and pain-relieving properties and may help regulate menstrual cycles. It can be consumed as tea or added to food as a spice.

Cinnamon: Cinnamon is believed to have anti-inflammatory and insulin-regulating properties and may help regulate menstrual cycles. It can be added to food or consumed as tea.

Turmeric: Turmeric is a powerful anti-inflammatory spice that may help regulate menstrual cycles. It can be added to food or consumed as a supplement.

Vitex: Vitex, also known as chasteberry, is a natural remedy that has been used for centuries to regulate menstrual cycles. It is believed to work by promoting hormonal balance and can be taken as a supplement.

Maca: Maca is a root vegetable that is commonly used as a natural remedy for menstrual irregularities. It is believed to work by promoting hormonal balance and can be consumed as a supplement or added to food.

Yoga and meditation: Stress can disrupt menstrual cycles, so practicing relaxation techniques such as yoga and meditation may help regulate menstrual cycles and promote hormonal balance.

Healthy diet and lifestyle: Eating a balanced diet, getting regular exercise, and avoiding tobacco and excessive alcohol can also help regulate menstrual cycles and promote hormonal balance.

Hot flashes:

Natural remedies such as black cohosh, evening primrose oil, and dong quai have been found to reduce the frequency and severity of hot flashes. Lifestyle changes such as staying cool, staying hydrated, and avoiding triggers (such as alcohol, caffeine, and spicy foods) can also help.

In addition to lifestyle changes, herbal remedies such as evening primrose oil, dong quai, and sage can also help alleviate hot flashes. Phytoestrogen-rich foods and lentils may also be helpful.

Here is a list of ways to alleviate your hot flashes:

Black cohosh: Black cohosh is a herb that is commonly used to alleviate hot flashes. It is believed to work by regulating hormone levels in the body.

Soy: Soy contains phytoestrogens, which are plant compounds that mimic the effects of estrogen in the body. Consuming soy products such as tofu or soy milk may help alleviate hot flashes.

Flaxseed: Flaxseed is rich in lignans, which are plant compounds that have estrogen-like effects in the body. Adding flaxseed to the diet may help alleviate hot flashes.

Red clover: Red clover is a herb that contains phytoestrogens and may help alleviate hot flashes.

Evening primrose oil: Evening primrose oil is rich in gamma-linolenic acid (GLA), which is an essential fatty acid that may help alleviate hot flashes.

Vitamin E: Vitamin E is an antioxidant that may help alleviate hot flashes. It can be consumed as a supplement or obtained from food sources such as nuts and seeds.

Mind-body techniques: Techniques such as deep breathing, yoga, and meditation can help alleviate hot flashes by reducing stress and promoting relaxation.

Cool drinks and clothing: Drinking cool liquids and wearing lightweight, breathable clothing can help alleviate hot flashes by lowering body temperature.

Night sweats:

Similar to hot flashes, natural remedies such as black cohosh, evening primrose oil, and dong quai can help reduce night sweats.

In addition to the herbal remedies mentioned above for hot flashes, valerian root and melatonin supplements can also help improve sleep quality and reduce night sweats.

Vaginal dryness:

Natural remedies such as vitamin E oil, coconut oil, and aloe vera gel can be used to alleviate vaginal dryness. Over-the-counter moisturizers or lubricants can also be used.

In addition to the natural remedies mentioned above, borage oil and sea buckthorn oil are other options that can help improve vaginal moisture and elasticity. Listed below are a few oils that can be used ofr vaginal dryness:

Coconut oil: Coconut oil is a natural lubricant that can be used to alleviate vaginal dryness. It is also antibacterial and antifungal, which can help prevent infection.

Olive oil: Olive oil is another natural lubricant that can be used to alleviate vaginal dryness. It is rich in antioxidants, which can help promote vaginal health.

Almond oil: Almond oil is a natural emollient that can help moisturize the vaginal tissues and alleviate dryness.

Vitamin E oil: Vitamin E oil is a powerful antioxidant that can help promote vaginal health and alleviate dryness.

Jojoba oil: Jojoba oil is a natural lubricant that can be used to alleviate vaginal dryness. It is also rich in nutrients and antioxidants, which can help promote vaginal health.

Evening primrose oil: Evening primrose oil is rich in gamma-linolenic acid (GLA), which can help promote vaginal health and alleviate dryness.

Grapeseed oil: Grapeseed oil is a natural lubricant that can be used to alleviate vaginal dryness. It is also rich in antioxidants, which can help promote vaginal health.

When using oils for vaginal dryness, it is important to choose pure, organic oils that are free of additives and preservatives. It is also recommended to test a small amount of oil on the skin before use to check for any allergic reactions or irritation.

It is important to note that while natural oils can help alleviate vaginal dryness, they do not address the underlying cause of the dryness

Decreased libido:

Natural remedies such as maca root, ginseng, and ginkgo biloba can help improve libido. Counseling, therapy, and lifestyle changes can also be beneficial.

In addition to the natural remedies mentioned above, ashwagandha and the list below may also help improve sexual function and libido.

Maca: Maca is a root vegetable that is commonly used as a natural remedy for sexual dysfunction. It is believed to work by promoting hormonal balance and increasing blood flow to the genitals.

Tribulus terrestris: Tribulus terrestris is a herb that has been used for centuries to enhance sexual function. It is believed to work by increasing testosterone levels in the body.

Ginseng: Ginseng is a root that has been used for centuries to enhance sexual function. It is believed to work by improving circulation and reducing stress.

Ashwagandha: Ashwagandha is a herb that is commonly used to reduce stress and anxiety, which can have a positive impact on libido.

Zinc: Zinc is an essential mineral that plays a role in the production of testosterone. Consuming zinc-rich foods such as oysters, beef, and pumpkin seeds may help boost libido.

Vitamin D: Vitamin D is important for overall health, including sexual function. Spending time in the sun or taking a vitamin D supplement may help boost libido.

Exercise: Regular exercise can help boost libido by reducing stress, improving circulation, and increasing self-confidence.

Communication: Relationship issues can contribute to a decreased libido. Open communication with your partner can help resolve issues and improve sexual function.

Mood swings:

Natural remedies such as St. John's wort, black cohosh, and omega-3 fatty acids can help alleviate mood swings. Stress reduction techniques, such as meditation and yoga, can also be helpful.

In addition to the natural remedies mentioned above, saffron and kava kava have been found to be effective in improving mood and reducing anxiety.

St. John's Wort: St. John's Wort is a herb that has been used for centuries to alleviate symptoms of depression and anxiety, including mood swings.

Omega-3 fatty acids: Omega-3 fatty acids are important for brain health and may help alleviate mood swings. Consuming omega-3-rich foods such as fatty fish, flaxseeds, and chia seeds can be helpful.

B-complex vitamins: B vitamins, including B6 and B12, are important for mood regulation. Taking a B-complex supplement or consuming foods such as leafy greens, whole grains, and lean protein can be helpful.

Exercise: Regular exercise can help alleviate mood swings by reducing stress and releasing endorphins, which are natural mood-boosters.

Meditation and yoga: Mind-body practices such as meditation and yoga can help alleviate mood swings by reducing stress and promoting relaxation.

Sleep: Lack of sleep can contribute to mood swings. Practicing good sleep hygiene, such as avoiding electronic devices before bed and creating a relaxing bedtime routine, can be helpful.

Herbal teas: Herbal teas such as chamomile, passionflower, and lavender can help alleviate mood swings by promoting relaxation and reducing stress.

Depression:

Natural remedies such as saffron, and the list below may help alleviate depression. Counseling, therapy, and lifestyle changes can also be beneficial.

In addition to the natural remedies mentioned above, St. John's wort has been found to be effective in treating mild to moderate depression.

St. John's Wort: St. John's Wort is a herb that has been used for centuries to alleviate symptoms of depression. It is believed to work by increasing levels of serotonin, a neurotransmitter that is associated with mood regulation.

Omega-3 fatty acids: Omega-3 fatty acids are important for brain health and may help alleviate symptoms of depression. Consuming omega-3-rich foods such as fatty fish, flaxseeds, and chia seeds can be helpful.

B-complex vitamins: B vitamins, including B6 and B12, are important for mood regulation. Taking a B-complex supplement or consuming foods such as leafy greens, whole grains, and lean protein can be helpful.

Exercise: Regular exercise can help alleviate symptoms of depression by releasing endorphins, which are natural mood-boosters.

Meditation and yoga: Mind-body practices such as meditation and yoga can help alleviate symptoms of depression by reducing stress and promoting relaxation.

Saffron: Saffron is a spice that has been found to have antidepressant effects. It can be consumed as a supplement or added to food.

Acupuncture: Acupuncture is a traditional Chinese medicine technique that involves the insertion of needles into specific points on the body. It has been found to be effective for some people in alleviating symptoms of depression

It is important to note that while natural remedies can be effective for some people, they may not work for everyone. Individuals experiencing symptoms of depression should discuss treatment options with their healthcare provider to determine the underlying cause and the most appropriate course of treatment. In some cases, medication and/or therapy may be necessary to effectively manage symptoms of depression

Anxiety:

Natural remedies such as passionflower, valerian root, and lavender can help alleviate anxiety. Stress reduction techniques, such as meditation and yoga, can also be helpful.

In addition to the natural remedies mentioned above, passionflower and chamomile tea can also help alleviate anxiety symptoms.

Chamomile: Chamomile is a herb that has been found to have calming effects and may help alleviate symptoms of anxiety. It can be consumed as a tea or taken as a supplement.

Lavender: Lavender is a herb that has been found to have calming effects and may help alleviate symptoms of anxiety. It can be used as an essential oil, added to bathwater, or consumed as a tea.

Passionflower: Passionflower is a herb that has been found to have calming effects and may help alleviate symptoms of anxiety. It can be consumed as a tea or taken as a supplement.

Exercise: Regular exercise can help alleviate symptoms of anxiety by releasing endorphins, which are natural mood-boosters.

Meditation and yoga: Mind-body practices such as meditation and yoga can help alleviate symptoms of anxiety by reducing stress and promoting relaxation.

Valerian root: Valerian root is a herb that has been found to have calming effects and may help alleviate symptoms of anxiety. It can be consumed as a tea or taken as a supplement.

Omega-3 fatty acids: Omega-3 fatty acids are important for brain health and may help alleviate symptoms of anxiety. Consuming omega-3-rich foods such as fatty fish, flaxseeds, and chia seeds can be helpful.

It is important to note that while natural remedies can be effective for some people, they may not work for everyone. Individuals experiencing symptoms of anxiety should discuss treatment options with their healthcare provider to determine the underlying cause and the most appropriate course of treatment. In some cases, medication and/or therapy may be necessary to effectively manage symptoms of anxiety.

Insomnia:

Natural remedies such as valerian root, chamomile tea, and lavender can help improve sleep. Good sleep hygiene practices, such as keeping a consistent sleep schedule, avoiding caffeine and alcohol, and keeping the bedroom cool and quiet, can also be helpful.

In addition to the natural remedies mentioned above, lavender oil and magnesium supplements can also help improve sleep quality.

Melatonin: Melatonin is a hormone that is produced by the body to regulate sleep. Taking a melatonin supplement may help alleviate symptoms of insomnia.

Valerian root: Valerian root is an herb that has been found to have sedative effects and may help alleviate symptoms of insomnia. It can be consumed as tea or taken as a supplement.

Chamomile: Chamomile is an herb that has been found to have calming effects and may help alleviate symptoms of insomnia. It can be consumed as tea or taken as a supplement.

Lavender: Lavender is an herb that has been found to have calming effects and may help alleviate symptoms of insomnia. It can be used as an essential oil, added to bathwater, or consumed as tea.

Exercise: Regular exercise can help alleviate symptoms of insomnia by reducing stress and promoting relaxation.

Magnesium: Magnesium is an essential mineral that is important for sleep and relaxation. Taking a magnesium supplement or consuming magnesium-rich foods such as leafy greens, nuts, and seeds can be helpful.

Avoiding caffeine and alcohol: Caffeine and alcohol can disrupt sleep and contribute to insomnia. Avoiding these substances before bedtime can be helpful.

Fatigue:

Natural remedies such as iron supplements, vitamin B12, and CoQ10 can help alleviate fatigue. Exercise and a healthy diet can also be beneficial.

In addition to the natural remedies mentioned above, iron-rich foods such as spinach and lentils can help alleviate fatigue. See the above list below for more remedies for fatigue.

Getting enough sleep: Ensuring that you are getting enough sleep, and improving sleep quality by practicing good sleep hygiene, can be helpful in alleviating fatigue.

Regular exercise: Regular exercise can help increase energy levels and alleviate fatigue by boosting circulation and increasing endorphins.

Healthy diet: Eating a balanced diet that is rich in whole foods such as fruits, vegetables, lean protein, and whole grains can help alleviate fatigue by providing the body with necessary nutrients and reducing inflammation.

Stress reduction techniques: Practicing relaxation techniques such as meditation, yoga, and deep breathing can help alleviate fatigue by reducing stress and promoting relaxation.

Stay hydrated: Dehydration can contribute to fatigue, so staying well-hydrated by drinking plenty of water and avoiding sugary drinks can be helpful.

Herbal teas: Herbal teas such as green tea and ginseng tea can help alleviate fatigue by providing a natural energy boost.

Essential oils: Essential oils such as peppermint, eucalyptus, and lemon can help alleviate fatigue by providing a natural energy boost and promoting mental clarity.

Weight gain:

A healthy diet and regular exercise can help prevent weight gain during menopause. Supplements such as green tea extract, fiber supplements, and probiotics can also be beneficial.

In addition to the natural remedies mentioned above, green tea extract has been found to be effective in aiding weight loss and reducing belly fat. See list below.

Regular exercise: Regular exercise can help with weight management by boosting metabolism, building muscle, and burning calories.

Healthy diet: Eating a balanced diet that is rich in whole foods such as fruits, vegetables, lean protein, and whole grains can help with weight management by providing the body with necessary nutrients and reducing inflammation.

Portion control: Eating smaller, more frequent meals throughout the day can help with weight management by keeping metabolism active and reducing overeating.

Fiber-rich foods: Eating foods that are high in fiber, such as beans, whole grains, and vegetables, can help with weight management by promoting feelings of fullness and reducing calorie intake.

Drinking water: Drinking plenty of water can help with weight management by promoting hydration, reducing overeating, and boosting metabolism.

Herbal teas: Herbal teas such as green tea and oolong tea can help with weight management by promoting fat burning and reducing appetite.

Stress reduction techniques: Practicing relaxation techniques such as meditation, yoga, and deep breathing can help with weight management by reducing stress and promoting healthy habits

Bloating:

A healthy diet low in sodium and high in fiber can help reduce bloating. Supplements such as probiotics and digestive enzymes can also be helpful.

In addition to the natural remedies mentioned above, fennel seeds and ginger tea can also help alleviate bloating as well as the list below.

Probiotics: Probiotics are beneficial bacteria that can help improve gut health and alleviate bloating. They can be consumed as supplements or found in foods such as yogurt, kefir, and sauerkraut.

Fiber-rich foods: Eating foods that are high in fiber, such as beans, whole grains, and vegetables, can help alleviate bloating by promoting regular bowel movements and reducing constipation.

Peppermint: Peppermint is an herb that has been found to have anti-inflammatory effects and may help alleviate bloating. It can be consumed as tea or taken as a supplement.

Ginger: Ginger is an herb that has been found to have anti-inflammatory effects and may help alleviate bloating. It can be consumed as tea or added to food.

Fennel: Fennel is a herb that has been found to have anti-inflammatory effects and may help alleviate bloating. It can be consumed as a tea or added to food.

Dandelion tea: Dandelion tea is a herbal tea that has been found to have diuretic effects and may help alleviate bloating.

Stay hydrated: Drinking plenty of water can help alleviate bloating by promoting hydration and reducing water retention.

Headaches:

Natural remedies such as feverfew, magnesium, and vitamin B2 can help alleviate headaches. Avoiding triggers, such as certain foods and stress, can also be beneficial.

In addition to the natural remedies mentioned above, peppermint oil and butterbur supplements can also help alleviate headaches.

Hydration: Drinking plenty of water can help alleviate headaches by promoting hydration and reducing dehydration-related headaches.

Magnesium: Magnesium is an essential mineral that is important for muscle and nerve function. Taking a magnesium supplement or consuming magnesium-rich foods such as leafy greens, nuts, and seeds can be helpful in alleviating headaches.

Ginger: Ginger is a herb that has been found to have anti-inflammatory effects and may help alleviate headaches. It can be consumed as a tea or added to food.

Peppermint: Peppermint is a herb that has been found to have anti-inflammatory effects and may help alleviate headaches. It can be consumed as a tea or applied as an essential oil to the temples.

Relaxation techniques: Practicing relaxation techniques such as meditation, deep breathing, and yoga can help alleviate headaches by reducing stress and promoting relaxation.

Essential oils: Essential oils such as lavender, eucalyptus, and chamomile can help alleviate headaches by promoting relaxation and reducing stress.

Acupressure: Acupressure is a traditional Chinese medicine technique that involves applying pressure to specific points on the body. It has been found to be effective in alleviating headaches for some people.

Joint pain:

Natural remedies such as omega-3 fatty acids, turmeric, and ginger can help alleviate joint pain. Exercise and maintaining a healthy weight can also be beneficial.

In addition to the natural remedies mentioned above, devil's claw and willow bark supplements can also help alleviate joint pain.

Turmeric: Turmeric is a spice that contains curcumin, a compound that has anti-inflammatory effects. Consuming turmeric or taking a curcumin supplement may help alleviate joint pain.

Omega-3 fatty acids: Omega-3 fatty acids are important for reducing inflammation and can be found in fatty fish such as salmon, mackerel, and sardines, as well as in flaxseeds and chia seeds.

Exercise: Low-impact exercise such as walking, swimming, and cycling can help alleviate joint pain by promoting circulation and reducing inflammation.

Heat therapy: Applying heat to the affected joint, such as with a hot water bottle or warm towel, can help alleviate joint pain and stiffness.

Cold therapy: Applying cold to the affected joint, such as with an ice pack, can help reduce inflammation and alleviate joint pain.

Massage: Massage can help alleviate joint pain by promoting circulation, reducing inflammation, and promoting relaxation.

Acupuncture: Acupuncture is a traditional Chinese medicine technique that involves inserting thin needles into specific points on the body. It has been found to be effective in alleviating joint pain for some people.

Muscle tension:

Natural remedies such as magnesium, epsom salt baths, and massage can help alleviate muscle tension. Exercise and maintaining good posture can also be helpful.

In addition to the natural remedies mentioned above see the list below.

Stretching: Regular stretching can help alleviate muscle tension by promoting flexibility and reducing muscle tightness.

Massage: Massage can help alleviate muscle tension by promoting circulation, reducing inflammation, and promoting relaxation.

Heat therapy: Applying heat to the affected area, such as with a hot water bottle or warm towel, can help alleviate muscle tension and stiffness.

Cold therapy: Applying cold to the affected area, such as with an ice pack, can help reduce inflammation and alleviate muscle tension.

Magnesium: Magnesium is an essential mineral that is important for muscle and nerve function. Taking a magnesium supplement or consuming magnesium-rich foods such as leafy greens, nuts, and seeds can be helpful in alleviating muscle tension.

Essential oils: Essential oils such as lavender, peppermint, and eucalyptus can help alleviate muscle tension by promoting relaxation and reducing stress.

Acupuncture: Acupuncture is a traditional Chinese medicine technique that involves inserting thin needles into specific points on the body. It has been found to be effective in alleviating muscle tension for some people

Memory lapses:

Natural remedies such as ginkgo biloba, omega-3 fatty acids, and vitamin E can help improve memory. Keeping mentally active and engaged can also be beneficial.

In addition to the natural remedies mentioned above, ginseng and bacopa supplements can also help improve memory. See also list below.

Ginkgo Biloba: Ginkgo Biloba is an herb that has been found to have cognitive-enhancing effects and may help alleviate memory lapses. It can be consumed as a supplement.

Omega-3 fatty acids: Omega-3 fatty acids are important for brain function and can be found in fatty fish such as salmon, mackerel, and sardines, as well as in flaxseeds and chia seeds.

Exercise: Regular exercise can help improve cognitive function by promoting circulation and reducing inflammation.

Healthy diet: Eating a balanced diet that is rich in whole foods such as fruits, vegetables, lean protein, and whole grains can help with memory and cognitive function by providing the body with necessary nutrients.

Stay hydrated: Dehydration can contribute to cognitive impairment, so staying well-hydrated by drinking plenty of water and avoiding sugary drinks can be helpful.

Herbal teas: Herbal teas such as green tea and rosemary tea can help improve cognitive function by promoting mental alertness and reducing oxidative stress.

Sleep: Getting enough sleep is important for cognitive function and memory consolidation. Ensuring that you are getting enough sleep, and improving sleep quality by practicing good sleep hygiene, can be helpful in alleviating memory lapses.

Difficulty concentrating:

Natural remedies such as ginkgo biloba, omega-3 fatty acids, and vitamin E can help improve concentration. Keeping mentally active and engaged can also be beneficial.

In addition to the natural remedies mentioned above, the following list can help with concentration.

Exercise: Regular exercise can help improve cognitive function and reduce stress, both of which can contribute to difficulty concentrating.

Sleep: Getting enough sleep is important for cognitive function and mental clarity. Ensuring that you are getting enough sleep, and improving sleep quality by practicing good sleep hygiene, can be helpful in alleviating difficulty concentrating.

Mindfulness practices: Practicing mindfulness techniques such as meditation, deep breathing, and yoga can help alleviate difficulty concentrating by reducing stress and promoting relaxation.

Hydration: Drinking plenty of water can help alleviate difficulty concentrating by promoting hydration and reducing dehydration-related symptoms.

Healthy diet: Eating a balanced diet that is rich in whole foods such as fruits, vegetables, lean protein, and whole grains can help with cognitive function by providing the body with necessary nutrients.

Caffeine: Caffeine is a natural stimulant that can help improve mental alertness and concentration. However, it is important to consume caffeine in moderation and not rely on it as a long-term solution.

Essential oils: Essential oils such as peppermint, rosemary, and lemon can help alleviate difficulty concentrating by promoting mental alertness and reducing stress

Brain fog:

Natural remedies such as ginkgo biloba, omega-3 fatty acids, and vitamin E can help alleviate brain fog. Keeping mentally active and engaged can also be beneficial.

In addition to the natural remedies mentioned above, ashwagandha and rhodiola supplements can also help alleviate brain fog. See also list below.

Exercise: Regular exercise can help improve cognitive function and reduce stress, both of which can contribute to brain fog.

Sleep: Getting enough sleep is important for cognitive function and mental clarity. Ensuring that you are getting enough sleep, and improving sleep quality by practicing good sleep hygiene, can be helpful in alleviating brain fog.

Hydration: Drinking plenty of water can help alleviate brain fog by promoting hydration and reducing dehydration-related symptoms.

Healthy diet: Eating a balanced diet that is rich in whole foods such as fruits, vegetables, lean protein, and whole grains can help with cognitive function by providing the body with necessary nutrients.

Mindfulness practices: Practicing mindfulness techniques such as meditation, deep breathing, and yoga can help alleviate brain fog by reducing stress and promoting relaxation.

Herbal remedies: Certain herbs such as ginseng, ginkgo biloba, and bacopa have been found to have cognitive-enhancing effects and may help alleviate brain fog. They can be consumed as supplements or added to food.

Essential oils: Essential oils such as peppermint, rosemary, and lemon can help alleviate brain fog by promoting mental alertness and reducing stress.

Hair loss or thinning:

Natural remedies such as biotin, zinc, and iron supplements can help improve hair health and reduce hair loss. A healthy diet and proper hair care can also be helpful.

In addition to the natural remedies mentioned above, saw palmetto supplements and pumpkin seed oil have been found to be effective in reducing hair loss and promoting hair growth.

Scalp massage: Massaging the scalp can help improve circulation to the hair follicles, which can promote hair growth and reduce hair loss.

Aloe vera: Aloe vera contains enzymes that can help promote hair growth and reduce hair loss. It can be applied topically to the scalp and hair.

Essential oils: Essential oils such as rosemary, lavender, and peppermint can help promote hair growth and reduce hair loss by improving circulation and stimulating hair follicles. They can be added to carrier oils such as coconut or jojoba oil and applied topically to the scalp and hair.

Nutrient-rich diet: Eating a balanced diet that is rich in vitamins and minerals such as biotin, iron, and zinc can help promote healthy hair growth and reduce hair loss.

Herbal supplements: Certain herbs such as saw palmetto, stinging nettle, and ginseng have been found to be effective in reducing hair loss and promoting hair growth. They can be consumed as supplements. Stress reduction: Reducing stress through practices such as meditation, yoga, and deep breathing can help reduce hair loss and promote hair growth.

Onion juice: Onion juice contains sulfur, which can help improve circulation to the hair follicles and promote hair growth. It can be applied topically to the scalp and hair

Dry skin:

Natural remedies such as coconut oil, vitamin E oil, and aloe vera gel can be used to alleviate dry skin. A healthy diet and staying hydrated can also be helpful.

In addition to the natural remedies mentioned above, hyaluronic acid supplements and shea butter can also help improve skin moisture and hydration.

Coconut oil: Coconut oil is a natural moisturizer that can help alleviate dry skin. It can be applied topically to the skin as a moisturizer.

Oatmeal: Oatmeal can help soothe dry, itchy skin by reducing inflammation and promoting hydration. It can be added to a warm bath or used in a homemade scrub.

Honey: Honey is a natural humectant that can help retain moisture in the skin. It can be added to a warm bath or applied topically as a mask.

Aloe vera: Aloe vera contains enzymes that can help soothe and hydrate dry skin. It can be applied topically to the skin as a moisturizer.

Hydration: Drinking plenty of water can help hydrate the skin from the inside out, which can help alleviate dry skin.

Humidifiers: Using a humidifier in the home can help add moisture to the air, which can help alleviate dry skin.

Avoiding harsh products: Avoiding harsh soaps and other products that can strip the skin of its natural oils can help alleviate dry skin

Acne:

Natural remedies such as tea tree oil, witch hazel, and apple cider vinegar can help alleviate acne. A healthy diet and proper skin care can also be beneficial.

In addition to the natural remedies mentioned above, zinc supplements and tea tree oil can also help reduce acne inflammation and improve skin texture.

Tea tree oil: Tea tree oil has antimicrobial properties that can help kill bacteria and reduce inflammation. It can be applied topically to the skin as a spot treatment.

Aloe vera: Aloe vera contains enzymes that can help reduce inflammation and soothe irritated skin. It can be applied topically to the skin as a moisturizer or mask.

Honey: Honey has antimicrobial properties that can help kill bacteria and reduce inflammation. It can be applied topically to the skin as a mask.

Apple cider vinegar: Apple cider vinegar can help balance the skin's pH and reduce inflammation. It can be diluted with water and applied topically to the skin as a toner.

Zinc: Zinc is an essential mineral that can help reduce inflammation and promote wound healing. It can be consumed as a supplement or applied topically to the skin as a cream.

Probiotics: Probiotics can help balance the bacteria in the gut, which can have a positive effect on the skin. They can be consumed as a supplement or found in fermented foods such as kimchi and sauerkraut.

Healthy diet: Eating a balanced diet that is rich in whole foods such as fruits, vegetables, lean protein, and whole grains can help promote healthy skin and reduce inflammation.

Brittle nails:

Natural remedies such as biotin, zinc, and iron supplements can help improve nail health and reduce brittleness. A healthy diet and proper nail care can also be helpful.

In addition to the natural remedies mentioned above, silica supplements and biotin can also help improve nail strength and reduce brittleness.

Biotin: Biotin is a B vitamin that is important for healthy nails. Consuming biotin-rich foods such as eggs, nuts, and sweet potatoes, or taking biotin supplements, can help improve nail health.

Vitamin E: Vitamin E is an antioxidant that can help improve nail strength and prevent breakage. It can be consumed as a supplement or applied topically to the nails.

Coconut oil: Coconut oil is a natural moisturizer that can help hydrate and strengthen brittle nails. It can be applied topically to the nails as a moisturizer.

Olive oil: Olive oil is rich in nutrients and can help strengthen and moisturize brittle nails. It can be applied topically to the nails as a moisturizer.

Horsetail: Horsetail is an herb that is rich in minerals such as silica, which can help improve nail strength and health. It can be consumed as tea or taken as a supplement.

Avoiding harsh chemicals: Avoiding harsh chemicals such as acetone and formaldehyde, which are often found in nail products, can help alleviate brittle nails.

Hydration: Drinking plenty of water can help keep the nails hydrated and prevent brittleness.

Breast tenderness:

Natural remedies such as evening primrose oil, flaxseed oil, and vitamin E can help alleviate breast tenderness.

In addition to the natural remedies mentioned above, flaxseed supplements and evening primrose oil can also help alleviate breast tenderness.

Supportive bra: Wearing a supportive bra can help reduce breast movement and alleviate breast tenderness.

Heat therapy: Applying a warm compress to the breasts can help reduce inflammation and alleviate breast tenderness.

Massage: Massaging the breasts can help improve circulation and reduce breast tenderness.

Vitamin E: Vitamin E is an antioxidant that can help reduce inflammation and alleviate breast tenderness. It can be consumed as a supplement or applied topically to the breasts.

Flaxseed: Flaxseed contains lignans, which can help balance hormones and reduce breast tenderness. It can be consumed as a supplement or added to foods such as smoothies and yogurt.

Avoiding caffeine: Caffeine can contribute to breast tenderness, so avoiding or reducing caffeine intake can be helpful.

Omega-3 fatty acids: Omega-3 fatty acids can help reduce inflammation and alleviate breast tenderness. They can be consumed as a supplement or found in foods such as fatty fish, flaxseed, and walnuts

Itchy skin:

Natural remedies such as oatmeal baths, aloe vera gel, and chamomile tea can be used to alleviate itchy skin. Avoiding harsh soaps and staying hydrated can also be helpful.

In addition to the natural remedies mentioned above, calendula cream and colloidal oatmeal baths can also help alleviate itchy skin.

Oatmeal: Oatmeal can help soothe and hydrate itchy skin by reducing inflammation. It can be added to a warm bath or used in a homemade scrub.

Aloe vera: Aloe vera contains enzymes that can help reduce inflammation and soothe irritated skin. It can be applied topically to the skin as a moisturizer or mask.

Apple cider vinegar: Apple cider vinegar can help balance the skin's pH and reduce itching. It can be diluted with water and applied topically to the skin as a toner.

Coconut oil: Coconut oil is a natural moisturizer that can help alleviate dry, itchy skin. It can be applied topically to the skin as a moisturizer.

Tea tree oil: Tea tree oil has antimicrobial properties that can help reduce itching and prevent infection. It can be applied topically to the skin as a spot treatment.

Calendula: Calendula has anti-inflammatory properties that can help reduce itching and promote healing. It can be applied topically to the skin as a cream or oil.

Hydration: Drinking plenty of water can help hydrate the skin from the inside out, which can help alleviate itching.

Allergies:

Natural remedies such as quercetin, stinging nettle, and butterbur can help alleviate allergies. Avoiding triggers, such as environmental allergens and certain foods, can also be beneficial.

In addition to the natural remedies mentioned above, quercetin supplements and nettle tea can also help alleviate allergy symptoms.

Quercetin: Quercetin is a flavonoid that has antihistamine and anti-inflammatory properties. It can be found in foods such as apples, onions, and green tea, or taken as a supplement.

Probiotics: Probiotics can help support a healthy immune system and reduce inflammation. They can be consumed as a supplement or found in fermented foods such as yogurt and sauerkraut.

Vitamin C: Vitamin C is an antioxidant that can help reduce inflammation and support a healthy immune system. It can be found in foods such as citrus fruits, bell peppers, and strawberries, or taken as a supplement.

Neti pot: A neti pot can help alleviate allergy symptoms by flushing out irritants and allergens from the nasal passages. It involves using a saline solution to rinse the nasal passages.

Honey: Honey contains pollen and can help desensitize the immune system to allergens. It is important to note that honey should not be given to infants under one year of age.

Steam inhalation: Steam inhalation can help alleviate congestion and reduce inflammation. It involves inhaling steam from a bowl of hot water or using a humidifier.

Essential oils: Essential oils such as lavender and peppermint can help reduce inflammation and alleviate allergy symptoms. They can be diffused or applied topically (diluted with a carrier oil).

Dry eyes:

Natural remedies such as omega-3 fatty acids and flaxseed oil can help alleviate dry eyes. Using a humidifier and avoiding prolonged screen time can also be helpful.

In addition to the natural remedies mentioned above, omega-3 fatty acid supplements and warm compresses can also help alleviate dry eyes.

Omega-3 fatty acids: Omega-3 fatty acids can help reduce inflammation and improve tear production. They can be consumed as a supplement or found in foods such as fatty fish, flaxseed, and chia seeds.

Warm compress: A warm compress can help stimulate tear production and reduce inflammation. It involves applying a warm, damp cloth to the closed eyes for several minutes.

Blinking exercises: Blinking exercises can help stimulate tear production and prevent dry eyes. It involves taking breaks throughout the day to blink several times in succession.

Hydration: Drinking plenty of water can help keep the eyes hydrated and prevent dryness.

Humidifiers: Using a humidifier in the home or workplace can help add moisture to the air, which can help alleviate dry eyes.

Eye massages: Massaging the eyelids can help stimulate tear production and alleviate dry eyes. It involves gently massaging the eyelids in a circular motion.

Rose water: Rose water has anti-inflammatory properties that can help reduce eye irritation and dryness. It can be applied topically to the eyes using a cotton pad.

Vision changes:

Natural remedies such as omega-3 fatty acids, lutein, and zeaxanthin can help support eye health and reduce vision changes. Protecting the eyes from UV rays and taking regular breaks from screens can also be beneficial.

Bilberry: Bilberry is a plant that is rich in antioxidants and can help improve night vision and reduce eye fatigue. It can be consumed as a supplement or found in foods such as berries.

Vitamin A: Vitamin A is important for healthy vision and can help reduce the risk of certain eye conditions. It can be found in foods such as sweet potatoes, carrots, and spinach, or taken as a supplement.

Eye exercises: Eye exercises can help strengthen the eye muscles and improve vision. They can include focusing on distant objects, tracing letters with the eyes, and moving the eyes in circles.

Hydration: Drinking plenty of water can help keep the eyes hydrated and prevent dryness, which can contribute to vision changes.

Anti-inflammatory foods: Consuming foods that are rich in anti-inflammatory nutrients such as omega-3 fatty acids and vitamin C can help reduce inflammation and improve vision. Foods such as fatty fish, nuts, and citrus fruits can be beneficial.

Resting the eyes: Resting the eyes can help alleviate eye strain and prevent further vision changes. It involves taking breaks throughout the day to close the eyes or look away from the screen.

Tinnitus:

Natural remedies such as ginkgo biloba, magnesium, and zinc can help alleviate tinnitus. Avoiding loud noises and reducing stress can also be helpful.

In addition to the natural remedies mentioned above, zinc supplements and acupuncture can also help alleviate tinnitus symptoms, including:

Magnesium: Magnesium can help improve blood flow and reduce inflammation, which can help alleviate tinnitus symptoms. It can be consumed as a supplement or found in foods such as nuts, seeds, and leafy green vegetables.

Zinc: Zinc can help improve immune function and reduce inflammation, which can help alleviate tinnitus symptoms. It can be consumed as a supplement or found in foods such as oysters, beef, and lentils.

Ginkgo biloba: Ginkgo biloba is an herb that can help improve circulation and reduce inflammation, which can help alleviate tinnitus symptoms. It can be consumed as a supplement.

Acupuncture: Acupuncture can help improve blood flow and reduce inflammation, which can help alleviate tinnitus symptoms. It involves the insertion of thin needles into specific points on the body.

Sound therapy: Sound therapy can help alleviate tinnitus symptoms by providing external sounds that can mask the internal sounds. It can involve using white noise machines, fans, or other devices that produce soothing sounds.

Meditation and relaxation techniques: Meditation and relaxation techniques can help reduce stress and improve circulation, which can help alleviate tinnitus symptoms. Techniques such as deep breathing, progressive muscle relaxation, and yoga can be helpful.

Dizziness:

Natural remedies such as ginger, ginkgo biloba, and vitamin D can help alleviate dizziness. Keeping hydrated and avoiding sudden movements can also be beneficial.

In addition to the natural remedies mentioned above, ginger supplements and acupuncture can also help alleviate dizziness.

Ginger: Ginger can help reduce inflammation and improve circulation, which can help alleviate dizziness. It can be consumed as tea, added to meals, or taken as a supplement.

Hydration: Drinking plenty of water can help prevent dehydration, which can contribute to dizziness.

Breathing exercises: Breathing exercises can help reduce stress and improve oxygen flow, which can help alleviate dizziness. Techniques such as deep breathing and diaphragmatic breathing can be helpful.

Vitamin D: Vitamin D is important for maintaining healthy bones and muscles, which can help prevent falls and alleviate dizziness. It can be found in foods such as fatty fish, egg yolks, and fortified foods, or taken as a supplement.

Exercise: Regular exercise can help improve circulation and reduce stress, which can help alleviate dizziness. Low-impact exercises such as walking, swimming, and yoga can be beneficial.

Salt: Consuming a small amount of salt can help raise blood pressure and alleviate dizziness. It is important to note that individuals with high blood pressure should consult with their healthcare provider before increasing salt intake.

Avoiding triggers: Avoiding triggers such as bright lights, loud noises, and certain foods can help alleviate dizziness.

Vertigo:

Natural remedies such as ginger, ginkgo biloba, and vitamin D can help alleviate vertigo. Keeping hydrated and avoiding sudden movements can also be beneficial.

In addition to the natural remedies mentioned above, acupuncture and vestibular rehabilitation can also help alleviate vertigo.

Ginger: Ginger can help reduce inflammation and improve circulation, which can help alleviate vertigo. It can be consumed as a tea, added to meals, or taken as a supplement.

Vitamin D: Vitamin D is important for maintaining healthy bones and muscles, which can help prevent falls and alleviate vertigo. It can be found in foods such as fatty fish, egg yolks, and fortified foods, or taken as a supplement.

Hydration: Drinking plenty of water can help prevent dehydration, which can contribute to vertigo.

Acupuncture: Acupuncture can help improve blood flow and reduce inflammation, which can help alleviate vertigo. It involves the insertion of thin needles into specific points on the body.

Breathing exercises: Breathing exercises can help reduce stress and improve oxygen flow, which can help alleviate vertigo. Techniques such as deep breathing and diaphragmatic breathing can be helpful.

Avoiding triggers: Avoiding triggers such as bright lights, loud noises, and certain foods can help alleviate vertigo.

Essential oils: Essential oils such as lavender and peppermint can help reduce stress and alleviate vertigo symptoms. They can be diffused or applied topically (diluted with a carrier oil).

Heart palpitations:

Natural remedies such as magnesium, hawthorn, and coenzyme Q10 can help alleviate heart palpitations. Reducing caffeine and alcohol consumption and managing stress can also be helpful.

In addition to the natural remedies mentioned above, magnesium supplements and hibiscus tea can also help alleviate heart palpitations.

Deep breathing: Deep breathing can help reduce stress and anxiety, which can contribute to heart palpitations. Techniques such as diaphragmatic breathing and box breathing can be helpful.

Magnesium: Magnesium can help regulate heart rhythm and reduce stress, which can alleviate heart palpitations. It can be consumed as a supplement or found in foods such as nuts, seeds, and leafy green vegetables.

Hydration: Drinking plenty of water can help prevent dehydration, which can contribute to heart palpitations.

Exercise: Regular exercise can help improve cardiovascular health and reduce stress, which can alleviate heart palpitations. Low-impact exercises such as walking, swimming, and yoga can be beneficial.

Caffeine reduction: Caffeine can contribute to heart palpitations, so reducing or eliminating caffeine intake can be helpful.

Herbal remedies: Herbal remedies such as hawthorn, valerian root, and passionflower can help regulate heart rhythm and reduce stress. They can be consumed as teas or taken as supplements.

Meditation and relaxation techniques: Meditation and relaxation techniques can help reduce stress and anxiety, which can contribute to heart palpitations. Techniques such as deep breathing, progressive muscle relaxation, and yoga can be helpful

High blood pressure:

Natural remedies such as garlic, hibiscus tea, and omega-3 fatty acids can help lower blood pressure. Maintaining a healthy weight and exercising regularly can also be beneficial.

In addition to the natural remedies mentioned above, hawthorn supplements and celery juice can also help lower blood pressure.

Regular exercise: Regular exercise can help lower blood pressure and improve overall cardiovascular health. Aim for at least 30 minutes of moderate-intensity exercise per day, such as brisk walking, cycling, or swimming.

Healthy diet: Eating a diet rich in fruits, vegetables, whole grains, and lean protein sources can help lower blood pressure. Limiting salt intake and avoiding processed and high-fat foods can also be beneficial.

Weight management: Maintaining a healthy weight can help lower blood pressure. Losing even a small amount of weight can make a significant difference.

Stress management: Chronic stress can contribute to high blood pressure, so finding ways to manage stress such as meditation, yoga, or deep breathing can be helpful.

Herbal remedies: Certain herbs such as garlic, hibiscus, and ginger can help lower blood pressure. They can be consumed as supplements or added to meals.

Magnesium: Magnesium can help regulate blood pressure and reduce stress. It can be consumed as a supplement or found in foods such as nuts, seeds, and leafy green vegetables.

Omega-3 fatty acids: Omega-3 fatty acids can help reduce inflammation and improve cardiovascular health. They can be found in fatty fish, nuts, and seeds or taken as a supplement.

Potassium: Potassium can help regulate blood pressure and reduce the effects of sodium on blood pressure. It can be found in foods such as bananas, avocados, and leafy green vegetables.

Hibiscus tea: Drinking hibiscus tea can help lower blood pressure. It is rich in antioxidants and can help improve overall cardiovascular health

Rapid heart rate:

Natural remedies such as magnesium, coenzyme Q10, and hawthorn can help alleviate a rapid heart rate. Reducing caffeine and alcohol consumption and managing stress can also be helpful.

In addition to the natural remedies mentioned above, valerian root supplements and deep breathing exercises can also help alleviate a rapid heart rate.

Deep breathing: Deep breathing exercises can help reduce stress and anxiety, which can contribute to a rapid heart rate. Techniques such as diaphragmatic breathing and box breathing can be helpful.

Hydration: Drinking plenty of water can help prevent dehydration, which can contribute to a rapid heart rate.

Magnesium: Magnesium can help regulate heart rhythm and reduce stress, which can alleviate a rapid heart rate. It can be consumed as a supplement or found in foods such as nuts, seeds, and leafy green vegetables.

Caffeine reduction: Caffeine can contribute to a rapid heart rate, so reducing or eliminating caffeine intake can be helpful.

Exercise: Regular exercise can help improve cardiovascular health and reduce stress, which can alleviate a rapid heart rate. Low-impact exercises such as walking, swimming, and yoga can be beneficial.

Herbal remedies: Certain herbs such as hawthorn, valerian root, and passionflower can help regulate heart rhythm and reduce stress. They can be consumed as teas or taken as supplements.

Meditation and relaxation techniques: Meditation and relaxation techniques can help reduce stress and anxiety, which can contribute to a rapid heart rate. Techniques such as deep breathing, progressive muscle relaxation, and yoga can be helpful.

Shortness of breath:

Natural remedies such as deep breathing exercises, magnesium, and coenzyme Q10 can help alleviate shortness of breath. Managing stress and avoiding triggers, such as pollution and allergens, can also be beneficial.

In addition to the natural remedies mentioned above, deep breathing exercises and pursed lip breathing can also help alleviate shortness of breath.

Deep breathing: Deep breathing exercises can help improve lung function and reduce stress, which can alleviate shortness of breath. Techniques such as diaphragmatic breathing and pursed lip breathing can be helpful.

Hydration: Drinking plenty of water can help prevent dehydration, which can contribute to shortness of breath.

Aromatherapy: Certain essential oils such as peppermint and eucalyptus can help open up airways and alleviate shortness of breath. They can be diffused or applied topically (diluted with a carrier oil).

Exercise: Regular exercise can help improve lung function and reduce stress, which can alleviate shortness of breath. Low-impact exercises such as walking, swimming, and yoga can be beneficial.

Herbal remedies: Certain herbs such as ginger and turmeric can help reduce inflammation and improve lung function. They can be consumed as supplements or added to meals.

Magnesium: Magnesium can help improve lung function and reduce stress, which can alleviate shortness of breath. It can be consumed as a supplement or found in foods such as nuts, seeds, and leafy green vegetables.

Meditation and relaxation techniques: Meditation and relaxation techniques can help reduce stress and anxiety, which can contribute to shortness of breath. Techniques such as deep breathing, progressive muscle relaxation, and yoga can be helpful.

Chest pain:

Natural remedies such as magnesium, hawthorn, and coenzyme Q10 can help alleviate chest pain. Managing stress and avoiding triggers, such as physical exertion and heavy meals, can also be helpful.

In addition to the natural remedies mentioned above, hawthorn supplements and nitric oxide- rich foods such as beets and leafy greens can also help alleviate chest pain.

Deep breathing: Deep breathing exercises can help reduce stress and anxiety, which can contribute to chest pain. Techniques such as diaphragmatic breathing and box breathing can be helpful.

Hydration: Drinking plenty of water can help prevent dehydration, which can contribute to chest pain.

Exercise: Regular exercise can help improve cardiovascular health and reduce stress, which can alleviate chest pain. Low-impact exercises such as walking, swimming, and yoga can be beneficial.

Herbal remedies: Certain herbs such as garlic and cayenne pepper can help improve circulation and alleviate chest pain. They can be consumed as supplements or added to meals.

Magnesium: Magnesium can help regulate heart rhythm and reduce stress, which can alleviate chest pain. It can be consumed as a supplement or found in foods such as nuts, seeds, and leafy green vegetables.

Meditation and relaxation techniques: Meditation and relaxation techniques can help reduce stress and anxiety, which can contribute to chest pain. Techniques such as deep breathing, progressive muscle relaxation, and yoga can be helpful.

Digestive problems:

Natural remedies such as probiotics, digestive enzymes, and peppermint tea can help alleviate digestive problems. Eating a healthy diet low in processed foods and high in fiber can also be beneficial.

In addition to the natural remedies mentioned above, peppermint oil supplements and artichoke leaf extract can also help alleviate digestive problems.

Probiotics: Probiotics can help restore healthy bacteria in the gut and alleviate digestive issues. They can be found in foods such as yogurt and fermented vegetables, or taken as a supplement.

Fiber: Consuming adequate amounts of fiber can help regulate digestion and alleviate constipation. Fiber-rich foods include fruits, vegetables, whole grains, and legumes.

Herbal remedies: Certain herbs such as ginger, peppermint, and fennel can help alleviate digestive issues such as bloating and nausea. They can be consumed as teas or taken as supplements.

Hydration: Drinking plenty of water can help prevent dehydration, which can contribute to constipation and other digestive issues.

Exercise: Regular exercise can help regulate digestion and alleviate constipation. Low-impact exercises such as walking, yoga, and cycling can be beneficial.

Stress management: Chronic stress can contribute to digestive issues, so finding ways to manage stress such as meditation, yoga, or deep breathing can be helpful.

Limiting trigger foods: Certain foods can trigger digestive issues, such as spicy or high-fat foods. Limiting or avoiding these foods can be helpful.

Constipation:

Natural remedies such as magnesium, fiber supplements, and probiotics can help alleviate constipation. Eating a healthy diet high in fiber and staying hydrated can also be helpful.

In addition to the natural remedies mentioned above, magnesium supplements and prunes can also help alleviate constipation.

Fiber: Consuming adequate amounts of fiber can help regulate digestion and alleviate constipation. Fiber-rich foods include fruits, vegetables, whole grains, and legumes.

Hydration: Drinking plenty of water can help prevent dehydration, which can contribute to constipation.

Probiotics: Probiotics can help restore healthy bacteria in the gut and alleviate constipation. They can be found in foods such as yogurt and fermented vegetables or taken as a supplement.

Exercise: Regular exercise can help regulate digestion and alleviate constipation. Low-impact exercises such as walking, yoga, and cycling can be beneficial.

Herbal remedies: Certain herbs such as senna, psyllium, and flaxseed can help alleviate constipation. They can be consumed as teas or taken as supplements.

Aloe vera: Aloe vera juice can help stimulate bowel movements and alleviate constipation.

Magnesium: Magnesium can help regulate bowel movements and alleviate constipation. It can be consumed as a supplement or found in foods such as nuts, seeds, and leafy green vegetables

Diarrhea:

Natural remedies such as probiotics, activated charcoal, and ginger can help alleviate diarrhea. Staying hydrated and avoiding trigger foods can also be beneficial.

In addition to the natural remedies mentioned above, activated charcoal supplements and glutamine can also help alleviate diarrhea.

Hydration: Drinking plenty of water and electrolyte-rich fluids such as coconut water and herbal teas can help prevent dehydration, which can accompany diarrhea.

Probiotics: Probiotics can help restore healthy bacteria in the gut and alleviate diarrhea. They can be found in foods such as yogurt and fermented vegetables or taken as a supplement.

Fiber: Consuming small amounts of soluble fiber such as oats, bananas, and sweet potatoes can help firm up stools and alleviate diarrhea.

Herbal remedies: Certain herbs such as ginger, peppermint, and chamomile can help alleviate diarrhea and reduce inflammation. They can be consumed as teas or taken as supplements.

Avoiding trigger foods: Certain foods such as high-fat or spicy foods can trigger diarrhea. Avoiding these foods can be helpful.

Rest: Resting and avoiding physical exertion can help alleviate diarrhea and reduce abdominal pain and cramping.

Zinc: Zinc can help reduce the duration and severity of diarrhea. It can be consumed as a supplement or found in foods such as lean meat, nuts, and seeds.

Incontinence:

Natural remedies such as pelvic floor exercises and bladder training can help improve bladder control. Maintaining a healthy weight and avoiding bladder irritants can also be helpful.

In addition to the natural remedies mentioned above, kegel exercises and bladder retraining can also help improve bladder control.

Pelvic floor exercises: Pelvic floor exercises, also known as Kegels, can help strengthen the muscles that control bladder and bowel function.

Hydration: Drinking plenty of water can help maintain bladder health and reduce the risk of urinary tract infections, which can contribute to incontinence.

Dietary changes: Consuming foods that are high in fiber can help regulate bowel movements and reduce the risk of fecal incontinence. Additionally, avoiding caffeine and alcohol can reduce the risk of urinary incontinence.

Bladder training: Bladder training involves gradually increasing the time between urination to help train the bladder to hold more urine.

Herbal remedies: Certain herbs such as horsetail and saw palmetto can help improve bladder function and reduce incontinence. They can be consumed as supplements or added to meals.

Acupuncture: Acupuncture can help regulate bladder function and reduce incontinence.

Biofeedback: Biofeedback involves using sensors to monitor muscle activity and provide feedback on how to better control bladder and bowel function.

Urinary tract infections:

Natural remedies such as cranberry supplements, probiotics, and D-mannose can help prevent and alleviate urinary tract infections. Drinking plenty of water and avoiding irritants can also be beneficial.

In addition to the natural remedies mentioned above, cranberry supplements and probiotics can also help prevent and alleviate urinary tract infections.

Hydration: Drinking plenty of water can help flush out bacteria and reduce the risk of UTIs.

Probiotics: Probiotics can help restore healthy bacteria in the urinary tract and reduce the risk of UTIs. They can be found in foods such as yogurt and fermented vegetables or taken as a supplement.

Cranberry: Cranberry contains compounds that can prevent bacteria from adhering to the urinary tract and reduce the risk of UTIs. It can be consumed as juice or taken as a supplement.

D-mannose: D-mannose is a type of sugar that can prevent bacteria from adhering to the urinary tract and reduce the risk of UTIs. It can be consumed as a supplement.

Herbal remedies: Certain herbs such as uva ursi and goldenseal can help reduce inflammation and infection in the urinary tract. They can be consumed as teas or taken as supplements.

Aromatherapy: Essential oils such as tea tree oil and oregano oil can help reduce inflammation and infection in the urinary tract. They can be used in aromatherapy or added to a warm bath.

Heat therapy: Applying a warm compress or taking a warm bath can help reduce inflammation and alleviate pain associated with UTIs.

Yeast infections:

Natural remedies such as probiotics, tea tree oil, and garlic can help alleviate yeast infections. Avoiding irritants and wearing loose-fitting clothing can also be helpful.

In addition to the natural remedies mentioned above, probiotics and tea tree oil suppositories can also help alleviate yeast infections.

Probiotics: Probiotics can help restore healthy bacteria in the gut and vagina and reduce the risk of yeast infections. They can be found in foods such as yogurt and fermented vegetables or taken as a supplement.

Garlic: Garlic contains compounds that have antifungal properties and can help alleviate yeast infections. It can be consumed raw or added to meals.

Tea tree oil: Tea tree oil has antifungal properties and can be applied topically to the affected area to alleviate yeast infections. However, it should be diluted before use.

Coconut oil: Coconut oil contains compounds that have antifungal properties and can help alleviate yeast infections. It can be applied topically to the affected area.

Boric acid: Boric acid has antifungal properties and can be used as a suppository to alleviate yeast infections. However, it should be used with caution and only under the guidance of a healthcare provider.

Apple cider vinegar: Apple cider vinegar can help balance the pH of the vagina and reduce the risk of yeast infections. It can be added to a warm bath or applied topically to the affected area.

Dietary changes: Avoiding sugary foods and refined carbohydrates can help reduce the risk of yeast infections, as these foods can contribute to the growth of Candida fungus.

Oral health problems:

Natural remedies such as xylitol gum, tea tree oil mouthwash, and oil pulling can help improve oral health. Eating a healthy diet low in sugar and staying hydrated can also be beneficial.

In addition to the natural remedies mentioned above, oil pulling with coconut oil and green tea supplements can also help improve oral health.

Good oral hygiene: Brushing and flossing regularly can help remove plaque and prevent tooth decay and gum disease.

Oil pulling: Swishing a tablespoon of coconut oil in the mouth for several minutes can help remove bacteria and promote oral health.

Saltwater rinse: Rinsing the mouth with warm saltwater can help reduce inflammation and alleviate discomfort associated with oral health problems.

Herbal remedies: Certain herbs such as sage and clove can help alleviate inflammation and discomfort associated with oral health problems. They can be consumed as teas or applied topically as a mouth rinse.

Probiotics: Probiotics can help restore healthy bacteria in the mouth and reduce the risk of oral health problems. They can be found in foods such as yogurt and fermented vegetables, or taken as a supplement.

Dietary changes: Consuming foods that are rich in vitamins and minerals, such as calcium and vitamin C, can help promote oral health and prevent oral health problems.

Gum disease:

Natural remedies such as aloe vera gel, tea tree oil, and coenzyme Q10 can help alleviate gum disease. Eating a healthy diet low in sugar and practicing good oral hygiene can also be helpful.

In addition to the natural remedies mentioned above, vitamin C supplements and probiotics can also help alleviate gum disease.

Herbal remedies: Certain herbs such as sage and peppermint can help alleviate inflammation and discomfort associated with gum disease. They can be consumed as teas or applied topically as a mouth rinse.

Probiotics: Probiotics can help restore healthy bacteria in the mouth and reduce the risk of gum disease. They can be found in foods such as yogurt and fermented vegetables or taken as a supplement.

Dietary changes: Consuming foods that are rich in vitamins and minerals, such as calcium and vitamin C, can help promote oral health and prevent gum disease.

Quitting smoking: Smoking can increase the risk of gum disease and inhibit the body's ability to heal from oral infections.

Tooth decay:

Natural remedies such as xylitol gum, fluoride toothpaste, and oil pulling can help prevent tooth decay. Eating a healthy diet low in sugar and practicing good oral hygiene can also be beneficial.

In addition to the natural remedies mentioned above, calcium supplements and xylitol gum can also help prevent tooth decay.

Good oral hygiene: Brushing and flossing regularly can help remove plaque and prevent the development of tooth decay.

Diet modifications: Consuming a diet that is low in sugar and processed foods can help reduce the risk of tooth decay. Additionally, consuming foods that are rich in vitamins and minerals, such as calcium and vitamin D, can help promote oral health and prevent tooth decay.

Xylitol: Xylitol is a natural sweetener that can help prevent the growth of bacteria in the mouth and reduce the risk of tooth decay. It can be consumed as a sugar substitute or added to oral care products.

Fluoride: Fluoride is a natural mineral that can help strengthen tooth enamel and prevent tooth decay. It can be found in certain foods and drinking water or added to oral care products.

Herbal remedies: Certain herbs such as neem and clove can help alleviate inflammation and discomfort associated with tooth decay. They can be consumed as teas or applied topically as a mouth rinse.

Oil pulling: Swishing a tablespoon of coconut oil in the mouth for several minutes can help remove bacteria and promote oral health, including preventing tooth decay.

Probiotics: Probiotics can help restore healthy bacteria in the mouth and reduce the risk of tooth decay. They can be found in foods such as yogurt and fermented vegetables or taken as a supplement.

Osteoporosis:

Natural remedies such as calcium, vitamin D, and weight-bearing exercise can help improve bone health and reduce the risk of osteoporosis. Avoiding smoking and excessive alcohol consumption can also be helpful.

In addition to the natural remedies mentioned above, vitamin K2 supplements and weight-bearing exercises such as weightlifting and hiking can also help improve bone health and reduce the risk of osteoporosis.

Adequate calcium and vitamin D intake: Consuming adequate amounts of calcium and vitamin D is essential for maintaining bone health and preventing osteoporosis. Calcium-rich foods include dairy products, leafy greens, and fortified foods, while vitamin D can be obtained from exposure to sunlight, fatty fish, and fortified foods.

Exercise: Regular weight-bearing exercise, such as walking, jogging, or strength training, can help maintain bone density and prevent osteoporosis.

Quitting smoking: Smoking can increase the risk of osteoporosis and inhibit the body's ability to heal from bone injuries.

Limiting alcohol consumption: Excessive alcohol consumption can increase the risk of osteoporosis and reduce bone density.

Herbal remedies: Certain herbs such as horsetail and red clover can help promote bone health and prevent osteoporosis. They can be consumed as teas or taken as supplements.

Magnesium: Magnesium is a mineral that can help promote bone health and prevent osteoporosis. It can be found in foods such as nuts, seeds, and whole grains, or taken as a supplement.

Omega-3 fatty acids: Omega-3 fatty acids can help promote bone health and reduce the risk of osteoporosis. They can be obtained from fatty fish, flaxseeds, and walnuts, or taken as a supplement.

Arthritis:

Natural remedies such as omega-3 fatty acids and turmeric, can help alleviate arthritis pain and inflammation. Exercise and maintaining a healthy weight can also be beneficial.

In addition to the natural remedies mentioned above, ginger tea and the list below can also help alleviate arthritis pain and inflammation.

Exercise: Regular low-impact exercise, such as walking, swimming, or yoga, can help reduce joint pain and stiffness, increase flexibility, and improve overall physical function.

Heat and cold therapy: Applying heat, such as with a warm towel or heating pad, or cold, such as with a cold compress or ice pack, can help reduce joint pain and stiffness.

Weight management: Maintaining a healthy weight can help reduce the stress on joints and alleviate arthritis symptoms.

Diet modifications: Consuming a diet that is rich in anti-inflammatory foods, such as fruits, vegetables, and fatty fish, and low in processed and fried foods can help reduce inflammation and alleviate arthritis symptoms.

Herbal remedies: Certain herbs such as turmeric, ginger, and Boswellia can help reduce inflammation and alleviate arthritis symptoms. They can be consumed as supplements or added to food.

Acupuncture: Acupuncture involves the insertion of thin needles into specific points on the body and has been shown to help reduce arthritis pain and inflammation.

Massage therapy: Massage therapy can help reduce muscle tension and joint stiffness associated with arthritis and promote relaxation.

Chronic fatigue syndrome:

Natural remedies such as CoQ10, B vitamins, and magnesium can help alleviate chronic fatigue syndrome. Managing stress and getting enough rest can also be helpful.

In addition to the natural remedies mentioned above ginseng and the list below can also help alleviate chronic fatigue syndrome.

Rest and sleep: Ensuring adequate rest and sleep is essential for managing CFS symptoms.

Diet modifications: Consuming a balanced and nutritious diet that is rich in whole foods, such as fruits, vegetables, whole grains, and lean protein, can help manage CFS symptoms.

Exercise: Regular low-impact exercise, such as walking, yoga, or tai chi, can help reduce fatigue and improve overall physical function.

Stress management: Managing stress through techniques such as deep breathing, meditation, and mindfulness can help reduce fatigue and improve overall well-being.

Herbal remedies: Certain herbs such as ashwagandha and licorice root can help reduce fatigue and improve energy levels. They can be consumed as supplements or added to food.

Vitamins and supplements: Certain vitamins and supplements such as B-complex vitamins, magnesium, and coenzyme Q10 can help reduce fatigue and improve energy levels.

Acupuncture: Acupuncture involves the insertion of thin needles into specific points on the body and has been shown to help reduce fatigue and improve energy levels in individuals with CFS.

Fibromyalgia:

Natural remedies such as magnesium, SAM-e, and acupuncture can help alleviate fibromyalgia symptoms. Exercise and managing stress can also be beneficial.

In addition to the natural remedies mentioned above, magnesium supplements and tai chi can also help alleviate fibromyalgia symptoms.

Exercise: Regular low-impact exercise, such as walking, swimming, or yoga, can help reduce pain and stiffness, increase flexibility, and improve overall physical function.

Stress management: Managing stress through techniques such as deep breathing, meditation, and mindfulness can help reduce pain and improve overall well-being.

Sleep hygiene: Ensuring adequate rest and sleep is essential for managing fibromyalgia symptoms. Establishing a regular sleep schedule and avoiding caffeine and alcohol can help improve sleep quality.

Diet modifications: Consuming a balanced and nutritious diet that is rich in whole foods, such as fruits, vegetables, whole grains, and lean protein, can help manage fibromyalgia symptoms.

Herbal remedies: Certain herbs such as St. John's Wort and valerian root can help reduce pain and improve sleep quality. They can be consumed as supplements or added to food.

Acupuncture: Acupuncture involves the insertion of thin needles into specific points on the body and has been shown to help reduce pain and improve overall well-being in individuals with fibromyalgia.

Massage therapy: Massage therapy can help reduce muscle tension and joint stiffness associated with fibromyalgia and promote relaxation.

Cancer (breast, ovarian, or endometrial):

*It is important to note that there is no single natural remedy that can prevent or cure breast or ovarian cancer. However, there are certain lifestyle modifications and natural remedies that may help reduce the risk of developing these cancers or improve the efficacy of medical treatments. These include:

Maintaining a healthy weight: Obesity and being overweight have been linked to an increased risk of breast and ovarian cancer. Maintaining a healthy weight through regular exercise and a balanced diet can help reduce the risk of developing these cancers.

Consuming a balanced and nutritious diet: A diet that is rich in fruits, vegetables, whole grains, and lean protein can help reduce the risk of developing breast and ovarian cancer. Additionally, certain foods such as cruciferous vegetables (broccoli, cauliflower, cabbage) and foods high in omega-3 fatty acids (fatty fish, flaxseeds, chia seeds) may have cancer-fighting properties.

Herbal remedies: Certain herbs such as turmeric, ginger, and green tea have been shown to have anti-cancer properties. They can be consumed as supplements or added to food.

Limiting alcohol consumption: Excessive alcohol consumption has been linked to an increased risk of breast and ovarian cancer. Limiting alcohol consumption to no more than one drink per day can help reduce the risk of developing these cancers.

Vitamin and mineral supplements: Certain vitamins and minerals such as vitamin D and calcium may help reduce the risk of developing breast and ovarian cancer. They can be obtained through diet or taken as supplements.

There are several herbs that have been studied for their potential anti-cancer properties. It's important to note that more research is needed to determine their effectiveness and safety in treating cancer. Here are some herbs that have been shown to have potential anti-cancer properties:

Turmeric: Curcumin, the active ingredient in turmeric, has been shown to have anti-inflammatory and anti-cancer properties. It has been studied for its potential to inhibit the growth of cancer cells and prevent the spread of cancer.

Ginger: Ginger contains compounds called gingerols and shogaols that have been shown to have anti-cancer properties. It has been studied for its potential to inhibit the growth of cancer cells and reduce inflammation.

Green tea: Green tea contains compounds called catechins that have been shown to have anti- cancer properties. It has been studied for its potential to inhibit the growth of cancer cells and reduce inflammation.

Milk thistle: Milk thistle contains a compound called silymarin that has been shown to have anti-cancer properties. It has been studied for its potential to inhibit the growth of cancer cells and protect healthy cells from damage.

Garlic: Garlic contains compounds such as allicin that have been shown to have anti-cancer properties. It has been studied for its potential to inhibit the growth of cancer cells and reduce inflammation.

*It's important to note that while these herbs have potential anti-cancer properties, they should not be used as a substitute for medical treatment. If you have been diagnosed with cancer, you should speak with your healthcare provider to determine the best course of treatment.

'Diabetes:

Natural remedies such as a healthy diet low in sugar and refined carbohydrates, regular exercise, and maintaining a healthy weight can help prevent and manage diabetes. Managing stress and getting enough rest can also be beneficial.

In addition to the natural remedies mentioned above, cinnamon supplements and chromium picolinate can also help improve blood sugar control and insulin sensitivity.

Diet modifications: Consuming a balanced and nutritious diet that is rich in whole foods, such as fruits, vegetables, whole grains, and lean protein, can help manage blood sugar levels.

Additionally, avoiding processed and high-sugar foods can help prevent spikes in blood sugar.

Exercise: Regular exercise can help manage blood sugar levels by increasing insulin sensitivity and improving glucose uptake by the muscles. Aim for at least 30 minutes of moderate- intensity exercise most days of the week.

Stress management: Managing stress through techniques such as deep breathing, meditation, and mindfulness can help reduce blood sugar levels and improve overall well-being.

Herbal remedies: Certain herbs such as ginseng, bitter melon, and cinnamon have been shown to have anti-diabetic properties. They can be consumed as supplements or added to food.

Vitamins and supplements: Certain vitamins and supplements such as magnesium, chromium, and alpha-lipoic acid can help improve blood sugar control and reduce inflammation.

Weight management: Maintaining a healthy weight through regular exercise and a balanced diet can help improve blood sugar control and reduce the risk of developing diabetes.

Menopause and Your Career

Menopause can have a significant impact on a woman's career in several ways. Here are some potential impacts of menopause on a woman's career:

Symptoms of menopause, such as hot flashes, mood swings, and fatigue, can affect a woman's ability to concentrate and perform at work.

Women may need to take time off work to manage menopause symptoms, which can impact their productivity and income.

Menopause can affect a woman's confidence and self-esteem, which may impact her ability to pursue career advancement opportunities.

Women may face discrimination or bias in the workplace due to their age or menopause status.

Women may feel pressured to hide their menopause symptoms in the workplace, which can add to their stress and impact their well-being.

However, there are also steps that women can take to manage the impact of menopause on their careers. These include:

Speaking with their healthcare provider to develop a plan for managing menopause symptoms.

Seeking support from colleagues, friends, or family members to help manage stress and emotional challenges.

Advocating for their needs in the workplace, such as requesting accommodations or time off as needed.

Seeking out career development opportunities that align with their goals and interests.

Finding ways to prioritize self-care, such as getting regular exercise, eating a balanced diet, and practicing stress management techniques.

Overall, menopause can be a challenging time for women in the workplace, but with the right support and strategies, women can continue to thrive in their careers during and after menopause.

Menopause and Relationships

Menopause can also have an impact on a woman's romantic and sexual relationships.

Along with symptoms like vaginal dryness, women may feel self-conscious or less attractive during menopause, which may impact their confidence in their relationships.

However, there are also ways to manage these challenges and maintain strong, healthy relationships during menopause. Here are some strategies:

Communicate openly and honestly with your partner about your symptoms and concerns.

Explore alternative forms of intimacy, such as touching, massage, or non-sexual physical contact.

Consider using vaginal moisturizers or lubricants to help manage vaginal dryness and discomfort during intercourse.

Seek support from a healthcare provider, therapist, or support group to manage mood swings or other emotional challenges.

Prioritize self-care, including getting adequate sleep, regular exercise, and a healthy diet, to help manage menopause symptoms and boost overall well-being.

Additionally, menopause can also have positive impacts on sexual relationships, such as increased communication or a deeper emotional connection.

It's important to remember that menopause is a normal and natural part of the aging process, and with the right support and strategies, women can maintain strong, healthy relationships during and after menopause.

Foods To Avoid During Menopause

Here are some examples of foods and liquids to avoid or limit during menopause:

Spicy foods:

Spices such as chili peppers, cayenne pepper, and black pepper can exacerbate hot flashes and night sweats in some women.

Alcohol:

All types of alcohol can worsen mood swings and disrupt sleep, but red wine may be particularly problematic due to its high levels of histamines and sulfites.

Caffeine:

Coffee, tea, energy drinks, and chocolate are all sources of caffeine that can cause irritability, nervousness, and sleep disturbances.

Sugar:

Foods high in added sugars, such as candy, soda, and baked goods, can cause energy crashes and mood swings.

Processed foods:

Processed foods such as fast food, frozen dinners, and packaged snacks are often high in unhealthy fats and sodium, which can worsen inflammation and contribute to weight gain.

It's important to note that everyone's body is different, and what triggers symptoms in one person may not have the same effect on another. Women may benefit from keeping a food diary to track which foods and drinks may exacerbate their symptoms, and work with a healthcare provider or registered dietitian to develop a nutrition plan that meets their individual needs.

Journalling During Menopause

Keeping a journal during menopause can be helpful in several ways. Here are some reasons why:

Tracking symptoms: Menopause can be a challenging time with many physical and emotional changes. Keeping a journal can help women track their symptoms and identify patterns or triggers that may be exacerbating their symptoms.

Identifying coping strategies: Women can use their journal to record which coping strategies, such as exercise or deep breathing, are most helpful for managing their symptoms. This can help them develop an effective self-care routine.

Documenting progress: Keeping a journal can help women see how far they've come in managing their menopause symptoms. It can be encouraging to look back and see that symptoms that were once overwhelming have become more manageable over time.

Expressing emotions: Menopause can be a time of intense emotions, including anxiety, depression, and anger. Writing in a journal can provide a safe space for women to express these feelings and work through them.

Improving communication with healthcare providers: By tracking their symptoms and experiences in a journal, women can provide more detailed information to their healthcare providers. This can help healthcare providers make more informed treatment decisions and provide more targeted support.

Overall, keeping a journal during menopause can be a powerful tool for self-care and managing symptoms. It can provide a sense of control during a time of change and help women feel empowered to take charge of their health and well-being.

How To Prepare for Bedtime During Menopause

Preparing for sleep during menopause can be a challenge, as hot flashes, night sweats, and other symptoms can interfere with a good night's rest. However, with some simple adjustments to your routine, you can improve your chances of getting a good night's sleep. Here are some tips for preparing for sleep during menopause:

Create a relaxing sleep environment: Make sure your bedroom is cool, quiet, and dark. Use earplugs or a white noise machine to block out any noise that may disrupt your sleep.

Practice good sleep hygiene: Establish a regular sleep routine by going to bed and waking up at the same time each day. Avoid caffeine, alcohol, and nicotine before bedtime, and limit your exposure to screens in the evening.

Exercise regularly: Regular exercise can improve sleep quality and reduce menopause symptoms. Aim for at least 30 minutes of moderate intensity exercise most days of the week.

Manage stress: Stress can exacerbate menopause symptoms and interfere with sleep. Practice relaxation techniques such as deep breathing, meditation, or yoga to help you manage stress.

Consider natural remedies: Some natural remedies, such as herbal teas or aromatherapy, may help promote relaxation and improve sleep. Talk to your healthcare provider about which remedies may be safe and effective for you.

Wear comfortable sleepwear: Choose breathable fabrics such as cotton or bamboo and avoid tight or restrictive clothing that may contribute to night sweats.

By taking steps to prepare for sleep during menopause, you can improve your chances of getting a good night's rest and feel more rested and refreshed each day.

What is HRT Hormone Replacement Therapy

Hormone replacement therapy (HRT) is a medical treatment that involves taking hormones to replace those that the body no longer produces naturally. In menopause, the ovaries stop producing estrogen and progesterone, which can lead to a range of symptoms such as hot flashes, night sweats, vaginal dryness, and mood changes. HRT is used to relieve these symptoms by supplementing the body with the hormones it needs.

HRT can be taken in several forms, including pills, patches, creams, gels, and vaginal rings. The hormones used in HRT can include estrogen alone, or a combination of estrogen and progesterone. The type of HRT used and the dosage will depend on individual factors, such as the severity of symptoms, medical history, and overall health.

The decision to take HRT is a personal one that should be made in consultation with a healthcare provider. Generally, women who are experiencing moderate to severe menopausal symptoms and who are in good health may benefit from HRT. Women who have had a hysterectomy may be able to take estrogen alone, while those who still have their uterus may need a combination of estrogen and progesterone to prevent the risk of endometrial cancer.

HRT can provide significant relief from menopausal symptoms and improve quality of life for many women. It can also have other potential health benefits, such as reducing the risk of osteoporosis and protecting against heart disease. However, HRT also carries some risks, such as an increased risk of blood clots, stroke, and breast cancer. Women who are considering HRT should talk to their healthcare provider about the potential benefits and risks, as well as alternative treatments that may be appropriate for their specific situation.

In summary, hormone replacement therapy is a medical treatment that involves supplementing the body with hormones that are no longer produced naturally during menopause. It can be an effective way to relieve menopausal symptoms and improve quality of life for many women, but it should be used carefully and with medical supervision. Women should work closely with their healthcare provider to determine whether HRT is appropriate for them and to monitor for any potential side effects.

Snoring and Menopause

Snoring is a common issue that can affect both men and women of all ages, but it may become more frequent during menopause. Menopause is a time when the body undergoes many hormonal changes, and these changes can lead to various sleep-related problems, including snoring.

One of the main reasons why menopausal women may snore more often is due to the decrease in estrogen levels. Estrogen plays a crucial role in maintaining the tone and strength of the muscles in the throat, including those that control breathing. As estrogen levels decline, these muscles can become weaker, leading to snoring.

Another reason why menopausal women may snore more is due to weight gain. Many women experience weight gain during menopause, which can lead to an increase in body fat, especially in the neck and throat area. This extra tissue can constrict the airways and make it more difficult to breathe, leading to snoring.

Other menopause-related symptoms, such as hot flashes and night sweats, can also disrupt sleep and contribute to snoring. Snoring can lead to poor quality sleep and daytime fatigue, which can further exacerbate other menopause-related symptoms.

If you are experiencing snoring during menopause, there are several things you can do to alleviate the problem. These include:

- Maintaining a healthy weight through a balanced diet and regular exercise
- Sleeping on your side, rather than on your back
- Avoiding alcohol and sedatives, which can relax the muscles in the throat and worsen snoring
- Using a humidifier in your bedroom to keep the air moist and reduce congestion
- Seeking treatment for underlying medical conditions, such as sleep apnea, that may be contributing to snoring

Here are some vitamins and supplements that may be helpful during menopause:

Calcium and Vitamin D:

Women's bone density tends to decrease during menopause, putting them at risk for osteoporosis. Calcium and vitamin D are essential for maintaining strong bones and may help reduce the risk of fractures.

Vitamin B12:

This vitamin is important for maintaining healthy nerve cells and producing red blood cells. Women may become deficient in vitamin B12 as they age, and deficiency can cause fatigue, weakness, and tingling sensations in the extremities.

Magnesium:

This mineral helps regulate muscle and nerve function and can help alleviate muscle tension, insomnia, and anxiety, which are common menopausal symptoms.

Vitamin E:

This vitamin has antioxidant properties and may help reduce hot flashes and night sweats in menopausal women.

Black Cohosh:

This herb has been traditionally used to alleviate menopausal symptoms, such as hot flashes and mood changes.

Soy Isoflavones:

Soy contains compounds called isoflavones, which can mimic the effects of estrogen in the body. Some studies have shown that soy isoflavones may help reduce the frequency and severity of hot flashes.

Probiotics:

These live bacteria can help promote a healthy gut microbiome, which can improve digestion and reduce inflammation in the body.

Omega-3 fatty acids:

These essential fatty acids have anti-inflammatory properties and can help improve heart health, reduce joint pain, and support brain function. Omega-3s are found in fatty fish, such as salmon and tuna, as well as in supplements like fish oil.

Vitamin C:

This antioxidant vitamin is important for immune function and can also help improve skin health and reduce the risk of cardiovascular disease.

Evening Primrose Oil:

This oil is derived from the seeds of the evening primrose plant and is rich in gamma-linolenic acid (GLA), an omega-6 fatty acid. GLA can help reduce inflammation and improve skin health, and evening primrose oil has been shown to alleviate some menopausal symptoms, such as hot flashes and breast tenderness.

Red Clover:

This herb contains isoflavones, which can mimic the effects of estrogen in the body and may help alleviate hot flashes and other menopausal symptoms.

Ginseng:

This herb has been used for centuries to improve energy, reduce stress, and improve overall well-being. Some studies have shown that ginseng may help alleviate menopausal symptoms, such as hot flashes and mood changes.

Vitamin K2:

This vitamin is important for bone health as it helps transport calcium to the bones, improving bone density. Vitamin K2 is found in fermented foods, such as natto and sauerkraut, as well as in supplements.

Melatonin:

This hormone is important for regulating the sleep-wake cycle and can help alleviate sleep disturbances, which are common during menopause.

St. John's Wort:

This herb has been traditionally used to treat depression and anxiety and may be helpful for women experiencing mood changes during menopause.

Ashwagandha:

This adaptogenic herb can help reduce stress and anxiety and may also improve sleep quality and support overall well-being.

Rhodiola Rosea:

This adaptogenic herb has been traditionally used to improve energy, reduce stress, and improve cognitive function.

Coenzyme Q10 (CoQ10):

This antioxidant compound is important for energy production and can help reduce fatigue and improve cardiovascular health.

Ginkgo Biloba:

This herb can help improve cognitive function, reduce anxiety, and alleviate some symptoms of menopause, such as hot flashes and mood changes.

Zinc:

This mineral is important for immune function, skin health, and hormone balance. Zinc deficiency can lead to a range of symptoms, including fatigue, hair loss, and weakened immune function.

Vitamin A:

This antioxidant vitamin is important for immune function, skin health, and vision. Vitamin A can also help improve bone density and reduce the risk of osteoporosis.

Vitamin B6:

This vitamin is important for maintaining healthy nerve and brain function, and may help alleviate symptoms such as mood swings, depression, and anxiety.

Vitamin B9 (Folic Acid):

This vitamin is important for healthy brain function and may also help reduce the risk of heart disease and stroke.

Vitamin B3 (Niacin):

This vitamin is important for energy production and can help reduce cholesterol levels and improve heart health.

Vitamin B5 (Pantothenic Acid):

This vitamin is important for healthy skin, hair, and nails, and may also help alleviate stress and anxiety.

Foods to eat during Menopause

Fruits and vegetables:

Fruits and vegetables are rich in antioxidants, vitamins, and minerals, which are important for overall health and well-being. Eating a variety of colorful fruits and vegetables can help reduce inflammation, improve immune function, and support healthy aging.

Whole grains: Whole grains, such as brown rice, quinoa, and oats, are rich in fiber, which can help regulate digestion and reduce the risk of chronic diseases such as heart disease, diabetes, and cancer.

Lean proteins:

Lean proteins, such as chicken, fish, tofu, and beans, are important for maintaining muscle mass and supporting bone health. They also provide important nutrients such as iron, zinc, and vitamin B12.

Calcium-rich foods:

Calcium is important for bone health, and women should aim to consume at least 1,000 mg of calcium per day during menopause. Good sources of calcium include dairy products, leafy greens such as kale and spinach, and fortified foods such as tofu and orange juice.

Foods rich in vitamin D:

Vitamin D is important for bone health and immune function, and many women do not get enough of it through diet alone. Good sources of vitamin D include fatty fish such as salmon, egg yolks, and fortified foods such as milk and cereal.

Healthy fats:

Healthy fats, such as those found in nuts, seeds, avocado, and fatty fish, are important for brain function, hormone balance, and reducing inflammation. Aim to incorporate a variety of healthy fats into your diet for optimal health.

Fermented foods:

Fermented foods, such as yogurt, kefir, kimchi, and sauerkraut, are rich in probiotics, which can help support digestive health and immune function. They may also help reduce inflammation and improve overall well-being.

Water:

Staying hydrated is important during menopause, as hormonal changes can lead to increased thirst and dryness. Aim to drink at least 8 cups of water per day, and consume hydrating foods such as fruits and vegetables.

Flaxseeds:

Flaxseeds are a good source of omega-3 fatty acids and lignans, which can help reduce inflammation and support hormonal balance. They can be added to smoothies, oatmeal, or salads for an extra nutrient boost.

Soy products:

Soy products, such as tofu, tempeh, and edamame, contain phytoestrogens, which can help alleviate some symptoms of menopause, such as hot flashes and mood changes. However, women with a history of estrogen-sensitive cancers should speak with their healthcare provider before incorporating soy into their diet.

Herbs and spices:

Herbs and spices, such as turmeric, ginger, and cinnamon, have anti-inflammatory properties and can help support overall health and well-being. They can be added to meals, teas, or smoothies for extra flavor and health benefits.

Dark chocolate:

Dark chocolate is a good source of antioxidants and may help improve mood and reduce stress. Aim for dark chocolate with at least 70% cacao for optimal health benefits.

Berries:

Berries are a good source of antioxidants and fiber, which can help reduce inflammation and support digestive health. They also contain compounds that may help improve cognitive function and reduce the risk of chronic diseases such as heart disease and cancer.

Nuts and seeds:

Nuts and seeds are a good source of healthy fats, protein, and fiber, which can help reduce inflammation and support overall health. They can be added to meals or eaten as a snack for a nutrient boost.

Herbal teas:

Herbal teas, such as chamomile, peppermint, and lavender, can help reduce stress, improve sleep quality, and alleviate some symptoms of menopause, such as hot flashes and mood changes. They can be consumed throughout the day as a soothing and healthful beverage.

Cruciferous vegetables:

Cruciferous vegetables, such as broccoli, cauliflower, and Brussels sprouts, contain compounds that may help reduce the risk of certain types of cancer. They are also rich in fiber and important nutrients such as vitamin C and vitamin K.

Avocado:

Avocado is a good source of healthy fats, fiber, and important nutrients such as vitamin K and potassium. It may also help reduce inflammation and support heart health.

Legumes:

Legumes, such as lentils, chickpeas, and black beans, are a good source of plant-based protein, fiber, and important nutrients such as iron and folate. They can be added to soups, salads, or used as a meat substitute for a healthful and filling meal.

Fermented soy products:

Fermented soy products, such as miso, natto, and tempeh, contain beneficial bacteria that can support gut health and boost immune function. They also provide protein, fiber, and important nutrients such as iron and calcium.

Seaweed:

Seaweed is a good source of iodine, which is important for thyroid function, as well as other important nutrients such as iron, calcium, and vitamin C. It can be added to soups, salads, or used as a wrap for a nutrient-dense meal.

Citrus fruits:

Citrus fruits, such as oranges, grapefruits, and lemons, are a good source of vitamin C, which is important for immune function and collagen production. They may also help reduce the risk of chronic diseases such as heart disease and cancer.

Sweet potatoes:

Sweet potatoes are a good source of fiber, vitamin A, and potassium, which can help support digestive health, vision, and heart health. They can be baked, roasted, or used as a substitute for regular potatoes for a nutrient-dense meal.

Green tea:

Green tea is a good source of antioxidants and may help reduce inflammation, improve brain function, and reduce the risk of chronic diseases such as heart disease and cancer.

It's important to note that a healthy and balanced diet should be individualized to meet each woman's unique needs and preferences.

Exercises to do during Menopause

Regular physical activity can be beneficial during menopause, as it can help reduce the risk of chronic diseases such as heart disease, diabetes, and osteoporosis. Here are some exercises to consider during menopause:

Cardiovascular exercise:

Cardiovascular exercise, such as walking, running, cycling, or swimming, can help improve heart health and reduce the risk of chronic diseases. Aim for at least 150 minutes of moderate-intensity exercise or 75 minutes of vigorous-intensity exercise per week.

Strength training:

Strength training, such as weightlifting or resistance band exercises, can help improve muscle strength and bone density. Aim for at least two days of strength training per week, targeting all major muscle groups.

Yoga or Pilates:

Yoga and Pilates can help improve flexibility, balance, and relaxation. They can also help reduce stress and alleviate some symptoms of menopause, such as hot flashes and mood changes.

Tai Chi:

Tai Chi is a gentle form of exercise that combines movement and meditation. It can help improve balance, flexibility, and relaxation.

Kegel exercises:

Kegel exercises can help strengthen the pelvic floor muscles, which can help alleviate urinary incontinence and improve sexual function. To do Kegel exercises, contract and hold the muscles used to stop urination for 5-10 seconds, then relax for 5-10 seconds. Repeat 10-15 times, three times per day.

Dancing:

Dancing is a fun and social way to get physical activity. It can improve cardiovascular health, flexibility, balance, and mood.

Swimming or water aerobics:

Swimming or water aerobics are low-impact exercises that can be easier on the joints. They can help improve cardiovascular health, muscle strength, and flexibility.

Hiking or nature walks:

Hiking or nature walks can be a great way to get physical activity while enjoying the outdoors. They can improve cardiovascular health, muscle strength, and mood.

It's important to speak with a healthcare provider before beginning a new exercise program, especially if you have any medical conditions or concerns.

Black Women and Menopause

Menopause is a natural biological process that affects all women, but the experience and symptoms of menopause can vary significantly among individuals. Some studies suggest that black women might experience menopause differently than women of other ethnicities due to a combination of genetic, cultural, and environmental factors. Here are some ways in which menopause might affect black women:

Age of onset:

Some studies suggest that black women may experience the onset of menopause slightly earlier than white women, although more research is needed to confirm this.

Symptoms:

Black women may report different types and severity of menopausal symptoms. For example, they may experience more frequent and severe hot flashes compared to white women. However, this can also vary significantly among individuals.

Cardiovascular health:

Black women are at a higher risk for developing cardiovascular diseases, such as hypertension and stroke, compared to women of other ethnicities. Menopause can exacerbate these risks due to the decline in estrogen levels, which have protective effects on cardiovascular health.

Mental health:

The menopausal transition can be a challenging time for many women, and black women may face unique stressors and social factors that can impact their mental health. Factors such as discrimination, income inequality, and limited access to healthcare resources can contribute to increased stress and poorer mental health outcomes.

Access to healthcare:

Black women may face barriers to accessing healthcare resources and receiving appropriate treatment for menopausal symptoms. These barriers can include economic limitations, cultural biases, and a lack of understanding or acknowledgement of their specific needs by healthcare providers.

It's important to note that these observations are general trends and that individual experiences can vary widely. Every woman's experience with menopause is unique, and factors such as genetics, lifestyle, and overall health can significantly impact the severity and duration of symptoms. It's crucial for women, regardless of their ethnicity, to have open conversations with their healthcare providers about their menopause experiences to ensure appropriate care and support.

References

North American Menopause Society. (2020). Menopause Guidebook. 9th Edition. The North American Menopause Society.
https://www.menopause.org/for-women/menopauseflashes/menopause-resource-center

Santoro, N., Epperson, C. N., & Mathews, S. B. (2015). Menopausal Symptoms and Their Management. Endocrinology and Metabolism Clinics of North America, 44(3), 497-515.
https://doi.org/10.1016/j.ecl.2015.05.001

National Institute on Aging. (2021). Menopause: Time for a Change. U.S. Department of Health and Human Services. https://www.nia.nih.gov/health/menopause

Harvard Medical School. (2019). Menopause: A Guide for Women and Those Who Love Them. Harvard Health Publishing.
https://www.health.harvard.edu/womens-health/menopause-a-guide-for-women-and-those-who-love-them

Minkin, M. J., & Wright, C. V. (2005). The Yale Guide to Women's Reproductive Health: From Menarche to Menopause. Yale University Press.

Greendale, G. A., & Sowers, M. (2013). The Menopause Transition. In J. S. Berek (Ed.), Berek and Novak's Gynecology (15th ed., pp. 1263-1311). Lippincott Williams & Wilkins.

Manson, J. E., & Bassuk, S. S. (2016). Hot Flashes, Hormones, and Your Health: Breakthrough Findings to Help You Sail Through Menopause. McGraw-Hill Education.

CPSIA information can be obtained
at www.ICGtesting.com
Printed in the USA
LVHW012321210423
745024LV00007B/139